MEDICAL TESTS YOU CAN DO YOURSELF

*More than 250 Simple, At-Home
Examinations and Observations*

Herbert Haessler, M.D., and
Raymond Harris

CB

CONTEMPORARY BOOKS

Library of Congress Cataloging-in-Publication Data

Haessler, Herbert.
    Medical tests you can do yourself : more than 250 simple, at-
home examinations and observations / Herbert Haessler and
Raymond Harris.
        p.   cm.
    Includes index.
    ISBN 0-8092-3038-0
    1. Diagnosis, Noninvasive.   2. Self-care, Health.   3. Medicine,
Popular.   I. Harris, Raymond.   II. Title.
RC71.6.H34   1997
616.02′4—dc21   97-14640
                                                    CIP

Cover design by Nick Panos
Interior design by City Desktop Productions

Published by Contemporary Books
An imprint of NTC/Contemporary Publishing Company
4255 West Touhy Avenue, Lincolnwood (Chicago), Illinois 60646-1975 U.S.A.
International Standard Book Number: 0-8092-3038-0
18   17   16   15   14   13   12   11   10   9   8   7   6   5   4   3   2   1

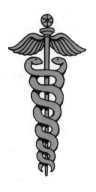

Contents

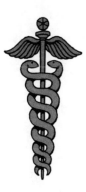

Acknowledgments

The authors extend enthusiastic thanks to certified nurse practitioner Diane Haessler, who reviewed the manuscript and provided valuable insights based on her grassroots work with people who are concerned about their health.

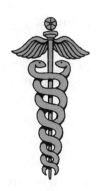

Introduction

Each time you see a new physician you are handed a clipboard with a long questionnaire attached. The doctor wants to know (in addition to what health insurance you carry) what diseases you have had, what operations, what medications you are taking, your immunization history, the health history of your parents and siblings, any allergies you know about, what your work is. The more you know, the better your treatment can be.

The next stop is the scale (you wish you hadn't worn those heavy shoes and you wonder if the nurse will think to deduct the weight of all the stuff in your pockets), your blood pressure and pulse are taken (you're sure these weren't as high before you walked into the examining room), and the nurse takes your temperature, probably with an electronic gizmo she inserts in your ear.

This is all vital information the doctor needs to become acquainted with your general condition and with any problems you may have. But so far, nothing very mysteri-

ous has happened that you couldn't have done yourself. And what is more, the information gathered probably isn't so accurate as you could have provided from the same tests performed at home under the everyday circumstances within which your body operates.

Blood pressure for many people rises as much as 10 to 20 percent as soon as they enter the examining room—what is called "white coat syndrome." This is the blood pressure that goes into your medical record, but if you have taken your blood pressure at home under a variety of real-life situations—with a perfectly good apparatus that costs less than $30—you can tell the doctor what your everyday average blood pressure is. The doctor will make a note of this and will know at once that he or she is dealing with an "activated" patient, someone who is aware of what is going on with his or her body. The doctor-patient relationship suddenly becomes a partnership between two people who can talk to one another on an equal plane about common problems they are trying to solve together.

As an activated patient you take an active interest in your body and its parts and in how they work together as an integrated whole. You come to know what looks and feels normal for you (normal is not the same for everyone) and to know what is not normal and requires the attention of your physician partner. When you report to your doctor for a checkup or because of illness, you can give the doctor an intelligent and informed appraisal of what's going on.

Chapter by chapter, *Medical Tests You Can Do Yourself* takes you through each of the body systems, showing how to do easy tests to determine how your body is functioning: checking your heart, lungs, and circulation; vision; hearing; the nervous system; the urinary system; the digestive process; bones, muscles, and joints; ears, nose, mouth, and throat; skin; and the reproductive systems. All of the tests described are noninvasive and safe to do yourself.

The equipment you need for home testing is inexpensive and easy to use: a fever thermometer, a blood-pressure cuff and stethoscope (less than $30 for both), a flashlight that you probably already have, and perhaps an inexpensive otoscope that is especially useful in families where there are a lot of earaches. And above all, you use your hands, your eyes, your ears, and a basic knowledge of your body and how it works.

Even a number of "lab" tests commonly thought of as being conducted only in a clinical setting are now available, inexpensively, on your drugstore shelf: urine tests, blood tests, tests for occult (hidden) bleeding, pregnancy tests, peak flow meters for people with respiratory ailments, AIDS tests, and many others.

Much of the mystery is going out of the doctor-patient relationship and most doctors are glad to see it go. It is being replaced by the intelligence, awareness, and common sense of informed patients who know their own bodies because they feel, see, and hear what is going on with that marvelous machine on a day-to-day basis.

Some examinations you do yourself can save your life. Many breast cancers in their early stages are still discovered by women who do their own testing. Melanoma, a particularly vicious and invasive skin cancer, is eminently curable in its early stages, and chances are it will be the patient who discovers the condition before the doctor does if the patient knows what he or she is looking for. An alert home examiner can spot the development of scoliosis in a young person, a spinal curvature that needs to be found early if treatment is to be successful. By doing simple home tests you can track your vision and discover subtle changes in the way you see that signal developing trouble that can be avoided with prompt medical attention.

While the training of health-care professionals, equipment, and medical procedures continue to improve, almost on a daily basis, health care itself has become less and less personalized than in years past. If you change jobs, if you move, or if your employer changes his or her health-insurance provider, you may not be able to keep the doctor you have come to know and who knows you. The new doctor, under time constraints from the new health plan, has to depend on you, to a large extent, to describe your symptoms and concerns completely.

Coming to the doctor armed with information about yourself is the best way to get the best treatment from your health-care provider. We hope this book will help you become an "activated" patient who will make the term *health maintenance* more meaningful in your family's quest for a longer, healthier life.

MEDICAL TESTS
YOU CAN DO
YOURSELF

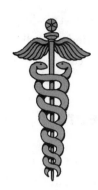

1

Examining and Testing Your Heart and Lungs

ore people die from heart and circulatory disease and malfunction than from any other cause, so it's no wonder that people worry more about their hearts than about any other part of the body. Worry, however, doesn't do your heart a bit of good. Anxiety about the heart can, and often does, cause needless incapacity in people who are actually well. What is better than worrying is getting to know your heart and treating it like the sturdy friend that it is.

The heart is a pump that moves blood throughout your entire body. Blood carries not only oxygen but all the essential nutrients to every organ, every muscle, every bone, every cell. It also carries waste products away from the cells that constitute body tissues. If they have no blood moving through them, many tissues die rather quickly. If the flow of blood to the brain is interrupted for any reason, irreversible damage occurs after five minutes.

So the heart is a very important organ. It is also a very well-designed and dependable organ that pumps along consistently, about seventy-two times a minute, one hundred thousand times a day, moving about two thousand gallons of blood without your being aware of it for the most part. And that's the way it should be. It will get along very nicely by itself without your worrying about it.

Getting to Know Your Heart

The heart is a very muscular organ. It is divided in half by a wall, or septum, that runs through the middle of the heart, inside, from top to bottom. Each side has two chambers, making four chambers in all—two auricles, or atria, that receive blood and two ventricles that pump it out again.

A highly efficient system of valves keeps blood flowing in the right direction, a rich network of blood vessels keeps the heart supplied with oxygen while it works, and a built-in pacemaker keeps the pumping action going at a regular rate. An automatic control system regulates the speed and strength of the pumping action in response to a complicated set of signals from various parts of the body. It all works so well that it couldn't be better if you had designed it yourself.

The two sides of the heart work in unison. The right side pumps blood through the lungs to collect oxygen. The oxygen-rich blood then returns to the left side of the heart and from there it is pumped to the rest of the body. The heart pumps blood by alternately squeezing to force blood into the blood vessels and then relaxing to allow the chambers to refill. The squeezing is called

the systolic action, or *systole* (sis'-tuh-lee), while the refilling phase is called the diastolic action, or *diastole* (di-ass'-tuh-lee).

Listening to Your Heart

Listening to heart sounds is one of the oldest medical tests. You can hear your heart beating quite easily with a simple instrument called a stethoscope. Before stethoscopes, doctors used a hollow tube to amplify the sound, and before that they just laid an ear against the patient's chest, which you can still do to hear the heart beat, though you don't have the clarity you can get with a stethoscope.

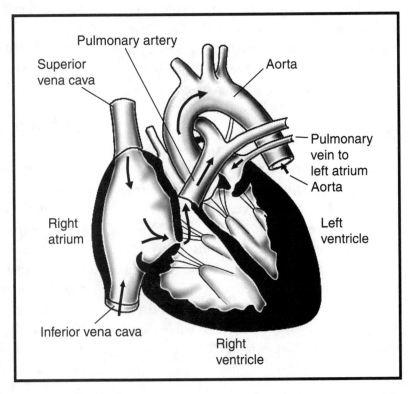

Diagram of the Heart with Direction of Blood Flow

Until rather recently, a stethoscope was a mysterious instrument to be used by medical personnel only. Left hanging around the neck or stuffed in the pocket of a white coat, it distinguished the professionals from the rest of the staff in a hospital. But stethoscopes became popular for home use once we began to realize the importance of individuals' monitoring their own blood pressure. They are now inexpensive and widely available at medical-supply stores, at some drugstores, and through advertisements in newspapers and magazines. And they are easy to use.

All stethoscopes consist of two hooked metal tubes that are fitted with earplugs which rest comfortably inside your ears. These metal tubes are attached to rubber or plastic tubing that is joined by a connector and then continues into a single tube which ends in either a flat or bell-shaped piece that is placed against the patient's chest to pick up sound.

Using a Stethoscope

1. Look at the earpieces of your stethoscope. Notice that the earplugs have a slant to them. Hold the stethoscope in front of you turned so that the curve or slant of the earplugs points slightly forward. Now place one of the earplugs in each ear. (You can rotate the earpieces of most stethoscopes so that they fit comfortably in your ears.)

2. To listen to your heart, place the flat or bell-shaped chest piece against your chest a little below the left nipple and just a bit toward the middle of your chest. Women should place the chest piece as close to the inside margin of the breast as possible. To hear your heart well, you must have good contact between your chest wall and the chest piece of the stethoscope. If the chest piece is rocking on a rib, move it slightly until it lies completely flat and firm against your skin. Women who have large breasts may be able to listen most easily by lifting the left breast with one hand and placing the chest piece up and under the breast as high as possible.

3. Listen carefully and you will hear your heart beating. It beats a little more often than once each second, about seventy-two times per minute. Each beat consists of two sounds that quickly follow each other. You should hear something that sounds like *lub-dub, lub-dub*. Move your stethoscope around a bit until the beat is loudest. The heart sounds will be slightly different in different parts of your chest. You should be able to hear your heart sounds from just below the inner edge of your collarbone on the left down to just above the next-to-last rib. You will usually be able to hear your heart more clearly near the central part of your chest than way out at the side.

Some people's heart sounds are much more easily heard than others. It is relatively easy to hear heart sounds in people with thin chest walls, and it is much more difficult to hear heart sounds in obese people. Except under unusual circumstances, however, difficulty in hearing heart sounds is not an indication of disease. If you have trouble finding an area where you can hear your heart sounds clearly, put your whole open hand over the lower part of your chest just under the left nipple, or underneath your breast in a line with the nipple. Sit up and lean forward. You should be able to feel your heart beating. The place where the heartbeat feels strongest is called the point of maximum impulse. Put the chest piece of the stethoscope here.

After you have found the various areas where you can hear your heart beating, listen carefully to the sounds. The two sounds come fairly close together: *lub-dub, lub-dub.* There should be a short space between the pairs of sounds where you hear little if anything. Each lub-dub pair represents a single heartbeat. The heart should beat regularly, anywhere from sixty to eighty times each minute. If you are an athlete or participate in an exercise program, your heart rate may be just a little under sixty beats per minute. And as you have surely noticed long before this, your heart beats faster when you exercise or if you are nervous.

When listening to the heart, you must listen carefully, first to the rhythm and regularity of the sounds and then to the quality of the sounds. Both are very important. The rhythm should be very regular—that is to say, the intervals between each lub-dub pair should be exactly the same. You won't be able to measure the intervals with a stopwatch, of course, but you will be able to hear whether the intervals are regular or irregular.

When listening to the rhythm, it is useful to count every time you hear a lub-dub pair. As you say the numbers—one, two,

three, four, five, etc.—you will be able to hear whether or not you are saying them in an absolutely regular sequence. The heart may speed up or slow down a bit from time to time, but it should continue to be regular. In some people, especially with children, the heart rate changes slightly with breathing. It tends to speed up just a bit when breathing in and then slows down when breathing out. This is normal and should not cause you to be concerned.

The heartbeat can be irregular in two ways. The first way is that an extra beat is inserted occasionally into the regular sequence. You hear the heart going lub-dub regularly and then all of a sudden an extra beat is inserted. Many people make these extra beats once every minute or two and in most cases they do not indicate heart disease. When you feel these extra beats, you may describe them as your heart jumping in your chest, or turning over, or even burping.

Sometimes you may feel these extra beats occurring in bursts and then nothing may happen again for hours. But if these extra beats become uncomfortable for you, they may need to be controlled with medication and it would be best to check with your doctor.

Almost everyone feels an irregular heartbeat from time to time. You might feel your heart skip a beat, or it might seem to race or palpitate, causing some discomfort and worry. Sometimes this happens when you are nervous or after an evening of too much of everything—especially too much coffee, liquor, and cigarettes. More often than not, these irregularities are harmless if they don't persist, but because they are disturbing, it's a good idea to have a doctor check into it—if only for the sake of reassurance and to hear once again that you should quit smoking and give up your stressful lifestyle.

Another kind of rhythm abnormality is an entirely uneven rhythm where the lub-dubs do not occur in any regular set beat. Sometimes this is associated with a very rapid heartbeat. The irregularities may occur for anywhere from five minutes to an hour or two and then revert to a normal regular beat. Or the irregular rhythm may be there all the time with the heart beating quite fast. These periods of irregularity may make you feel weak and washed out and they should be investigated and brought under control by your doctor.

Once you have determined that your heart rhythm is regular, you should then concentrate on the quality of the sounds. Most abnormal heart sounds are called *murmurs*. A murmur is a sort of blowing sound and occurs most frequently between the two major heart sounds—that is, between the lub and the dub. If you have a heart murmur, it may sound like lub-shss-dub, lub-shss-dub. But sometimes murmurs occur after the end of the second heart sound, giving a lub-dub-shss, lub-dub-shss.

If you find you have a heart murmur, this does not necessarily mean you have something wrong with your heart that needs immediate attention. The presence of a murmur only means there is something about the shape of your heart that does not allow the blood to flow smoothly through the heart chambers and valves that connect them, and you can be perfectly well and healthy living with a heart murmur. But

there are heart murmurs that sometimes indicate serious problems with heart valves and other internal structures of the heart, so the prudent thing to do if you discover a murmur is to have it checked out by your doctor. If the verdict is that it's nothing to worry about, then don't worry about it.

Taking Your Pulse

Each time the heart beats there is a corresponding impulse in major blood vessels throughout the body. At points where arteries come near the surface of the body, these impulses can be felt quite easily. Because the impulses correspond exactly with your heartbeat, if you want to determine how fast your heart is beating it is easier to feel for the impulses than to listen to the heart. This is what you do when you check your pulse.

You can find a pulse beat just below your inside ankle bone, in your temples, on either side of your Adam's apple, and at several other places around the body. But the most popular and accessible place to take a pulse is on the wrist just below the base of the thumb.

Except for stress tests and measures of physical condition during exercise, the pulse should be measured at rest. Have a watch or a clock handy that has an easy-to-see sweep second hand.

1. Turn one hand palm up and wrap the fingers of your other hand around the wrist from the back so that the tips of your fingers are touching the wrist where you are taking the pulse, just below the base of the thumb. Grasp the wrist firmly

without squeezing. By grasping with all your fingers, you should feel the throbbing pulse beat at once. If you just poke at your wrist with one finger, you may have to move it around a bit before you find a spot where the pulse can be felt distinctly. (Do not use your thumb to feel for the pulse. You can often feel a pulse in your thumb so that the pulse on pulse can be confusing, especially when you take the pulse of another person.)

2. When you take someone else's pulse, it will probably be easier for you if he or she turns his or her hand with the palm facing down, and then you can wrap

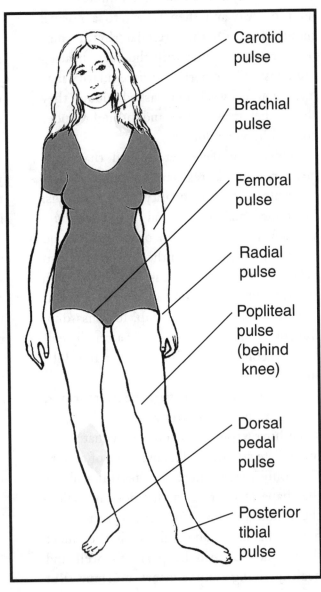

Carotid
pulse

Brachial
pulse

Femoral
pulse

Radial
pulse

Popliteal
pulse
(behind
knee)

Dorsal
pedal
pulse

Posterior
tibial
pulse

Pulse Points

your fingers around the top of the wrist, so that the tips of your fingers rest on the underside of the wrist at the base of the thumb.

3. Make sure you can feel the beat of the pulse under your fingertips, and as the second hand of your watch crosses a well-defined spot (twelve, three, six, and nine are favorite positions), begin to count pulse beats. Although you want the number of times the pulse beats in a minute, it isn't necessary to wait a whole minute to get your results. If the pulse feels steady and regular, count for just ten seconds and multiply by six. Or count for fifteen seconds and multiply by four.

4. If you want to take your pulse continuously during exercise, stop what you are doing and take your pulse quickly before it can slow down. If money is no object, you can buy a pulse-rate monitor at sporting-goods stores that monitors your pulse continuously. Some even sound an alarm when your pulse gets as high as you want it to be. They are priced from $100 to $150.

Many people have heard that a normal pulse rate when you are relaxed is seventy-two beats per minute. What is meant is that the *average* pulse rate of normally healthy people in our population is seventy-two beats per minute. Athletes and people in very good physical condition who exercise regularly will often have slow pulse rates, sometimes sixty or even lower when they are relaxed. Smok-

ers and people in poor physical condition tend to have higher pulse rates.

Exercise, of course, increases the pulse rate. A young athlete in good condition can tolerate a peak performance pulse of 150 without difficulty. The pulse rate also increases with anxiety, emotional upset, excitement, and sexual activity.

Pulse rates of small children can be normal when more than ninety beats per minute. But pulse rates that are above eighty may indicate a problem in adults. The pulse increases five to ten beats per minute for every degree of body temperature above what is normal for you. (The average normal is 98.6° F. Normal for you may be a little lower or a little higher.) So if your temperature is hovering around 101° F, your pulse rate may be as high as ninety-two.

Severe anemia, thyroid disease, and some infections all increase the pulse rate. If your resting pulse rate is regularly over eighty or at the most eighty-five beats per minute, you should bring this to the attention of your doctor.

A slower than normal pulse rate can occur in a few acute illnesses, but these are also associated with other much more obvious physical discomforts that would prompt you to seek the help of a physician. More often, people with acute illnesses have abnormally fast pulse rates. If your resting pulse rate rises and stays appreciably above what you have established as normal for you, or if your pulse is "normally" over eighty, you and your doctor should try to find out why. Irregular heart rhythms are also reflected in the pulse, and if you detect this happening frequently, or if you feel uncomfortable with periods of irregular pulse beat, check this out with your doctor, too.

Someone who has had a sudden heart attack, who is going into shock for some reason, or who has severe pain will usually have a very fast pulse rate. With someone who is acutely ill the quality of the pulse is often poor. It is not only rapid but is sometimes described as "thin" or "thready." This means that the beats are not very strong. Anyone who seems acutely ill and has a fast, thready pulse rate needs immediate medical attention.

Because "normal" can vary so widely among people, it is a good idea to know what your resting, relaxed pulse is when you are well. Then you will be in a position to observe deviations from what is normal for you. If you are in a gradually increasing physical-conditioning program, if you have learned to be less anxious, or if you have given up smoking, excess alcohol, and coffee, chances are good you will notice a decline in your normal pulse rate. It is not unusual, for instance, for a person to start with a pulse of eighty beats per minute and drop to fifty or sixty beats per minute after several months of regular exercise. Generally speaking, if you are also feeling well, this is just what the doctor ordered.

If you are in a program of regular, vigorous exercise and want to track the improvement in your pulse rate, you can use the following step test, but use it with caution.

The Two-Minute Step Test

Caution: The step test is equivalent to climbing six or seven flights of stairs at a fast pace. If you have been sedentary, if your exercise regimen has been spotty and less than vigorous and you are just beginning to exercise vigorously, if you have a heart problem, if you are recovering from an illness, or if you are over thirty-five and have not consulted with a doctor concerning your level of fitness, you should not do the step test.

1. Stand at the bottom of a stairway where there is a rail or bannister to help keep your balance if you need to. Step up onto the *second* step (skipping the first one) so that you are standing on it with both feet. Then step down, again bypassing the first step.

2. Repeat stepping on and off the second step this way for two minutes at the rate of thirty round trips a minute. You can have someone time you, or count as you exercise—one second up, one second down—and you will be at about the right speed.

3. At the end of two minutes of exercise, sit down and rest for two minutes.

4. After resting for two minutes take your pulse. Record the result and try again in about two weeks. If you exercise regularly and vigorously in the meantime, you should find your pulse gradually slowing down.

Recognizing Exercise-Induced Angina

Angina is pain resulting from the heart muscle not getting sufficient blood via the arteries that feed it, usually because one or more arteries are clogged and narrowed with fatty deposits called plaque. It can appear as pain in the center of the chest that is often described as feeling as if there were a heavy weight sitting on you. In describing the pain of angina, patients often hold a clenched fist against their chest to demonstrate an oppressive, squeezing sensation. Angina can also be more subtle, causing radiating pain to the neck, jaw, shoulder, and arms—particularly the left arm, although the right arm sometimes feels the pain, too. And a number of people simply report "funny feelings" in their chest, neck, jaw, and arms when they exercise.

If you are doing the step test, or any other exercise, and you experience chest pain or any of the other funny feelings, you must stop at once and sit down to rest. The same applies if chest pain occurs during stressful situations or after a meal. If the pain soon goes away when you rest, you should make an appointment to see your doctor at once to check it out. Tell the appointment secretary that you are experiencing chest pain when you exercise so that you get to see the doctor quickly. But if the pain persists, you may be having a heart attack and you must take steps to get to the hospital at once, preferably via your community ambulance service.

With modern diagnostic and treatment procedures, it isn't necessary to wait until you have a heart attack to do something about badly blocked arteries. It is unfortunate that many people in their forties, fifties, and sixties ignore their pains and funny feelings, unaware that they are living with one or more major heart arteries that are 90 percent blocked, until a sudden shutdown causes a massive heart attack that kills without warning.

Recognizing a Heart Attack

A heart attack is an extremely serious medical event; anyone having an attack must go to a hospital emergency room promptly to receive proper medical treatment. Time is very important because many people experiencing a heart attack will be eligible to be given medicines designed to dissolve a blood clot in an obstructed artery causing the attack and that will allow blood to flow once again to the affected area of the heart. These are commonly called clot-buster drugs, and they must be started as soon as possible after the onset of the heart attack to have a reasonably good chance of working.

A heart attack may manifest itself in very obvious ways—as when a person has sudden chest pain and falls over unconscious—or produce the more subtle symptoms of angina—pain in the chest, neck, jaw, and arms as described previously. Someone suffering a heart attack may also sweat profusely while feeling cold and clammy. Whatever the severity of the pain, your emergency medical service should be called (911 in most communities) for transportation to the hospital by people who know what to do if the symptoms worsen or become critical.

The milder the chest pain and the more the symptoms deviate from those described, the harder it is to be sure you are having a heart attack. Too many people, under the influence of television advertising, take a painkiller or an antacid tablet and wait for the pain to go away. If there is any question in your mind that what you are experiencing may be a heart attack, it is best to go to a hospital emergency room immediately. A heart attack doesn't go away, and if your attack is such that some heart muscle can be saved, it will most likely be saved in the first hour or so after the attack.

It is true that other things can produce pain that resembles a heart attack. Digestive problems as well as anything that happens to go awry with the complex systems of muscles, nerves, bones, connective tissue, and other organs in the upper half of your body can produce chest pain. Of all the people who go to a hospital emergency room complaining of chest pain, far less than half are found to have anything wrong with their hearts. And the usual reaction is to feel foolish for having caused a lot of people a lot of trouble and worry. Emergency-room doctors, however, recognize that most patients coming to the hospital with chest pain will not be having heart attacks, and the doctors would much rather that that be the case than that you stay at home with a potentially lethal condition.

Taking Your Blood Pressure

High blood pressure, also known as hypertension, has been shown to be so closely related to the incidence of heart attacks and strokes that it is known, quite appropriately, as "the silent killer." At any one time, as many as 23 million people in the United States have abnormally high blood pressure—and many of them don't even know it. Blood-pressure clinics are conducted with increasing frequency where people work, as projects of civic organizations, in drugstores and supermarkets, at senior centers, or anyplace where large numbers of people can

hear the word and be tested. It has become almost an evangelical movement.

While taking blood pressure was once reserved for the hospital and the doctor's office, people now are encouraged to keep close tabs on their own blood pressure. To measure your blood pressure you need your stethoscope and a blood-pressure cuff, officially named *sphygmomanometer* (sfig-moh-muh-nom'-i-ter). The name comes from the Greek word *sphygmus*, which is simply our old friend the pulse, and *meter*, which means measure.

Blood-pressure cuffs are readily available from medical-supply stores, from drugstores, and through mail-order advertisements in many popular magazines and catalogs. Increased interest in home testing has led to the development of new kinds of blood pressure–testing instruments, including one that provides an automatic digital readout, one that fits like a wristwatch, and one that attaches to your finger. Before you buy, though, make careful inquiries about guarantees of accuracy as you would when buying a camera, stereo components, or any other equipment and be sure you receive a set of instructions. If in doubt, ask your doctor or other health professionals about their preferences. Dial or mercury-column types of sphygmomanometers are the ones most generally used at the present time, and the ones generally acknowledged to be the most accurate, so these are the kinds we will discuss.

When your heart pumps, it pushes blood into the arteries throughout your body. As long as the heart keeps pumping, the flow of blood is continuous. The heart, however, pumps with an intermittent squeezing action. Each beat includes a squeeze that you can feel as a pulse. With each beat the blood pressure rises to a peak level, and between beats it falls to a lower level. The highest level the blood pressure reaches is called the *systolic pressure*. This occurs when the heart is in systole, or when it is in its squeezing phase. The lowest level the blood pressure reaches is called the *diastolic pressure*. This occurs in diastole, or when the heart is refilling.

Blood pressure is normally recorded as two numbers, such as 120 over 74 (generally written as 120/74). The first, or larger, of the two numbers is the systolic pressure; the second, or smaller, is the diastolic pressure. The units of measurement of blood pressure are millimeters of mercury, the same units used to measure the atmospheric, or barometric, pressure recorded in weather reports.

Normal systolic pressures in adults range from 110 to 145. Normal diastolic pressures range from 60 to 90. In someone who seems well and is able to be up and about, low blood pressure has relatively little significance except that it is infinitely better to have low blood pressure than high blood pressure. High blood pressure—that is, pressure above 145 over 90—is a dangerous disorder.

Both exercise and emotional tension can elevate blood pressure; relaxation and meditation techniques can often lower it. However, if your resting blood pressure is consistently above 145 over 90, you should consult your doctor promptly. It can't be emphasized too strongly that untreated high blood pressure is a dangerous disease that can eventually lead to a substantially shortened life because of either a heart attack or a stroke. And elevated blood pressure can be very effectively treated with several different medicines. It should be noted, too, that, contrary to common belief, high blood pressure is not reserved exclusively for older people. It is not uncommon for some young people to have badly elevated blood pressure that should be treated as soon as it is discovered.

How to Use a Blood-Pressure Cuff

The following procedure is the one you would use with a dial or mercury-column apparatus, the kind used in hospitals or in a doctor's office. It is a little awkward to use by yourself, although with a little practice most people can use it well and accurately. However, if you have difficulty or if gadgets intimidate you, you may want to work with a partner or buy a machine that automatically produces a digital readout.

1. Wrap the blood-pressure cuff snugly around your upper arm, just above the elbow joint. Put the earpieces of your stethoscope in your ears ready to use.

2. Tighten the thumbscrew at the base of the inflation bulb. Inflate the cuff by pumping the bulb until the dial shows about 200 millimeters of mercury. This will produce quite a hard squeeze on the upper arm.

3. Bend the arm just a little bit at the elbow and place the diaphragm of the stethoscope in the little cupped part on the inside of the elbow joint.

4. Release the air pressure from the cuff slowly by loosening the thumbscrew a little. Listen carefully with your stethoscope as the dial shows the pressure coming down.

5. As the pressure comes down, you will suddenly begin to hear thumping sounds in your stethoscope. These will be regular and uniform sounds, one thump for each heartbeat. Note the pressure at which you hear the very first thump. This is the systolic pressure.

6. Continue listening as you let pressure out of the cuff. Note the pressure at the point where you stop hearing the thumping sounds. This is the diastolic pressure.

7. Wait a few minutes and then reinflate the cuff and take the measurements again to be sure you have conducted the test accurately. You may get slightly different readings each time, but they should be within a few points of one another.

Because many things can affect your blood pressure, it is a good idea to keep careful notes of the time of day when you do your test and your activity immediately preceding the test (include such things as arguments, worry, and other tension-causing situations). If you are taking any drug or medicine, record the fact and tell what it is. When you begin testing, take your blood pressure at least three days in a row under quiet, peaceful circumstances; shortly after you wake up in the morning is an ideal time.

If the results you get are inconsistent or confusing, take your equipment to your doctor or another person who takes blood pressure frequently and professionally. Review your procedure and compare results with your equipment and with theirs. If there is a discrepancy in equipment, have it checked by your medical-equipment dealer.

If you are under a doctor's care for hypertension, follow his or her directions explicitly. You may be directed to take your blood pressure under a variety of circumstances or before and after using your medication.

There is an interesting experiment you can try to demonstrate the effect of stress on your blood pressure: Take your blood pressure when you have experienced stress—an argument, worry, a tough day at work. Then relax using a meditation or relaxation technique, if you know one, for half an hour or relax by listening to soothing (not hard-rock) music and take your blood pressure again. You will almost surely see a decline unless you have intractable high blood pressure or blood pressure that is normally quite low.

Respiratory Rate, Lung Capacity, and the Sounds of Breathing

The main function of the lungs is to provide oxygen for the entire body and to get rid of the waste we produce in respiration—carbon dioxide. Respiration is the process in which body cells take in oxygen that is carried to them by the blood and give up waste carbon dioxide that is formed as the cells produce energy and go about the business of their highly specialized functions. The waste carbon dioxide is carried to the lungs by the blood, where it is disposed of as you breathe out. The blood picks up fresh oxygen from air breathed in by the lungs and makes its next delivery to the cells. And so it goes for as long as you live.

When the body is called on to work harder, as happens when you exercise, a complicated set of signals starts the heart pumping faster and the lungs breathing faster to fulfill the demand from the cells for more oxygen. If, for some reason, either your heart or lungs can't keep pace with the demand, you will find your ability to exercise, climb stairs, or run for a bus severely limited.

Checking Your Respiratory Rate

One of the fundamental measures of bodily function is the respiratory rate. This is the number of times you breathe in and out in one minute. A normal rate varies between fourteen and twenty times per minute. As with the heart rate, both exercise and fever raise the respiratory rate. A disorder of your thyroid gland may also increase your respiratory rate a little. Fever increases the respiratory rate about four breaths per minute for every degree of fever above 98.6° F. It is important to have a record of your respiratory rate when you are well and rested so that you can tell if the rate has increased significantly during times of stress or illness.

It is difficult to check your own respiratory rate because you become self-conscious and tend to breathe either faster or slower than you might when you are not paying attention to it. That's why a nurse will probably watch your respiratory rate while you think she is still checking your pulse. So ask someone else to catch you unawares and record your respiratory rate for you.

1. Ask someone to observe your breathing over a short period of time while you are relaxed and occupied with something that is nonstressful.

2. The observer should count the number of breaths you take in just fifteen seconds, or thirty seconds at the most, so that you don't become aware that you are being checked.

3. Because you want your respiratory rate per minute, multiply a fifteen-second count by four, or a thirty-second count by two, just as you did when taking your pulse.

Listening to Breath Sounds

You can learn the way your lungs sound as they breathe in and out in the same way you learned how the heart sounds, by listening to them with your stethoscope. Absolutely normal breath sounds are just the smooth flow of air in and out. You might think of them as about the way your breathing sounds after running a bit. Abnormal breath sounds include wheezing, rhonchus, and rales.

Wheezing sounds (sometimes heard with the stethoscope as squeaks and whistles) may occur when the major breathing passages are narrowed or obstructed, as happens to people with asthma. A rhonchus (pronounced ron'-kus, plural rhonchi) is the rattling sound you hear when there is an accumulation of mucous in the major airways—something you hear in heavy smokers, people with bad colds, and some people with certain breathing-obstructive diseases. Rales make very fine crackling sounds. These are not very loud and sound a bit like tissue paper being crumpled up. These are usually heard when serious illness is present. Any abnormal collection of fluid in the lungs may cause rales. Pneumonia causes rales and lung congestion from heart failure also causes rales.

1. Place your stethoscope earplugs in your ears and place the chest piece firmly against your chest. Start on the right side of your chest, just below the nipple. Women should start just below the right breast.

2. Open your mouth and take a deep breath. Then blow the breath out slowly.

3. Breathe in and out slowly with your mouth open. You should be able to hear very soft breath sounds in and out each time you breathe. Normal breath sounds sound about the way your breath sounds after you have been running and are breathing hard.

4. Move the stethoscope around to various areas of your chest—up high, down low, around the sides, and around the back. You will notice that your doctor does most of his or her listening to your lungs

from the back. This is partly because the breath sounds are a bit louder from the back and partly because the heartbeat is not so loud in the back, making it easier to hear the sounds in the left lung. You will not be able to reach very much of your own back with a stethoscope, but go back as far as you can, or work with a partner.

If you have asthma, you may hear some abnormal breath sounds like little squeaks and whistles. During an asthma attack these squeaks and whistles become very apparent; but even when the asthma is not giving any trouble there may be a few squeaks and whistles anyway, which, in an asthmatic person, have little meaning. The sounds, however, do disappear in most people when their asthma is not causing trouble.

When you have a cold you may also hear some abnormal breath sounds. These are caused by mucous in the upper airways and generally have little significance. Heavy smokers may also hear some strange sounds caused by mucous accumulation.

The condition known as emphysema is an overexpansion of alveoli in the lungs—small air sacs where the exchange of oxygen and carbon dioxide takes place during respiration. The walls of the alveoli break down and this naturally decreases the ability of the lungs to do their job. The first symptom of emphysema is usually shortness of breath when exercising or simply when climbing a flight of stairs. People with emphysema may also have a chronic accumulation of mucous in the large airways with resulting rhonchi, the rattling sounds. But breath sounds may be entirely absent low down in the lungs where alveoli have been destroyed.

Of all breathing difficulties, emphysema is the most avoidable. In at least 90 percent of emphysema patients, the condition has been caused or made worse by smoking. Dusts and irritating fumes in the workplace can also contribute to emphysema, and a combination of smoking and exposure to irritating fumes is virtually a sure route to emphysema, severely limited activity, and early death. Any damage to the alveoli by smoking or other irritants is irreversible, a good reason for smokers to quit smoking as soon as they can to prevent further damage.

Pneumonia

There are many causes and many types of pneumonia, but basically it is an inflammation of the air cells in the lungs (alveoli) that results in an accumulation of fluid or pus in one or more lobes of the lungs. It can be brought on by the activity of bacteria, a virus, chemical irritation, or even inactivity as when someone is confined to bed for a long period of time. Pneumonia can range from something that is easily controlled by antibiotics to more intractable forms with high fatality rates. Pneumonias caused by viruses, known as viral pneumonias, do not respond to any antibiotics presently available and, therefore, can be particularly dangerous. People in a weakened condition are particularly susceptible to pneumonia that follows on the heels of flu or even a simple cold. Because so many forms of pneumonia are caused by a wide variety of organisms, it

is important that when pneumonia is found that the precise cause be determined so that appropriate treatment can be prescribed.

When a person is quite sick with a cold or flu, the question always arises whether or not a trip to the doctor is necessary to check for pneumonia. When pneumonia is present, you may hear the fine crackling sound of rales at the base of one or both lungs when you listen with your stethoscope. If you hear rales in an ill person, it may not be pneumonia but it is at the very least an indication that you should see the doctor and perhaps have a chest x-ray. Fever with chills, chest pain, a deep cough that produces copious sputum, and looking and feeling quite ill are all signs of possible pneumonia and you should see a doctor without delay.

Tuberculosis

As recently as the early part of the twentieth century, tuberculosis was a widespread killer, commonly known as consumption or the "white plague." Tuberculosis mainly attacks the lungs, but many other organs of the body may also be affected. There are two main kinds of tuberculosis: human, where the tuberculosis bacterium is spread by droplet infection (coughing, for example), and bovine, where the bacterium is passed from infected cows to humans drinking their milk. Bovine tuberculosis has virtually disappeared wherever pasteurization of milk is the rule. With the introduction of powerful antibiotics after 1950, the incidence of tuberculosis plummeted in developed countries, and sanitariums that used to treat the disease with sun, fresh air, and nourishing diet disappeared.

But while the incidence of human tuberculosis is way down from where it was fifty years ago, it is still a formidable threat in places where there are poor, crowded conditions—which includes a large part of the world and even the inner cities of highly developed societies. And as some strains of the tuberculosis bacteria have developed resistance to antibiotics, the incidence of new cases of tuberculosis is on the rise once again and it has become harder to treat.

Tuberculosis is not easily acquired by casual contact with an infected person. But prolonged contact (by health-care workers or family members) can lead to infection. Because tuberculosis in its early stages may not produce any symptoms, every adult should be tested for tuberculosis at least once. This is a skin test where a tuberculin material is injected under the skin. The test is positive if swelling or a small bump appears at the injection site after a few days. This is not available as a home test. Symptoms of tuberculosis include:

- Fatigue and weakness
- Weight loss
- Persistent fever
- Profuse sweating at night
- Blood in sputum
- Persistent coughing where chronic bronchitis has been ruled out

All these symptoms can be signs of other diseases, but they should be called to the attention of your doctor so that tuberculosis can be ruled out as a cause.

Hyperventilation Syndrome

Hyperventilation is a frightening event that brings a surprising number of people to hospital emergency rooms. It is usually a form of anxiety attack. Because they are anxious or for some other reason, these people begin to breathe more quickly than they ordinarily would. The result is that they overoxygenate the blood and blow out more carbon dioxide than they should be doing. This lowers the pH of the blood, which results in a feeling of numbness in the lips, lightheadedness and minor confusion, a tingling of the fingers of both hands, and a feeling of heaviness in the arms.

This is a typical scenario for hyperventilation syndrome. It's scary because the person who is hyperventilating has been upset to start with, and then with the symptoms he or she becomes more and more anxious, overbreathes more and more so that it becomes a self-perpetuating condition. Eventually, if this goes on for too long, a person may pass out. At this point, the person stops overbreathing, the body corrects itself, and he or she is soon OK.

Before a person gets to this point, however, a simple trick may help. Crumple a paper lunch bag to fit over the nose and mouth and have the person breathe into it. This allows some of the carbon dioxide to be rebreathed and helps correct the blood pH level and the hyperventilator will feel better.

Don't assume, however, that a person complaining of difficulty breathing is simply hyperventilating. If there is a history of heart disease or the symptoms of angina described earlier are present, your emergency medical service should be called.

Vital Capacity and Peak Air Flow

During normal breathing, you never completely fill the lungs with all the air you can breathe, and in breathing out you never completely empty your lungs of air. But if a doctor suspects that you have a breathing problem, he or she will likely check your vital capacity. This is the maximum amount of air that you can take into your lungs and then expel completely. Using an apparatus called a spirometer, the doctor asks you to take in as large a breath as you possibly can. Then you exhale as much air as you can into the spirometer. The reading measures peak air flow from your lungs and tells the doctor if your lungs can hold as much air as the average person of your age and size.

The spirometer is not a practical instrument for you to own, but there is a simple way to check your peak air flow called the match test.

The Match Test

1. Light an ordinary match and hold it at arm's length.

2. Take a deep breath and try to blow the match out. Be sure your aim is good, of course, and there should not be any stray winds or drafts to help you.

3. If you can blow the match out without difficulty, your peak air flow is probably normal. If you can't blow out the match, mention this to your doctor.

Peak Flow Meter

If you are under treatment for asthma, emphysema, or some other breathing problem, your doctor may want you to own a peak flow meter. This is a relatively inexpensive instrument ($20 to $50) and can be purchased in a medical-supply store and in many pharmacies. If you are a smoker and can't quit, a peak flow meter can furnish you with graphic evidence of how your vital capacity is declining over time.

The doctor will tell you what your expected peak flow is when you are doing well. If your peak air flow begins to fall from this expected level, it could signal trouble—the coming of an asthma attack or the worsening of emphysema, for example. If your peak air flow falls below 80 percent of what is expected of you, your doctor should be told. If your peak air flow falls to 50 percent or lower, this signals a medical alert and the doctor should be contacted at once. You will be given a chart or other information that shows what these percentages are for you.

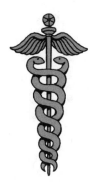

2

Knowing About Blood, Lymph, and Your Circulatory System

Blood is a complex body fluid that contains three distinct types of blood cells and a liquid component called plasma that not only carries the cells but virtually all the nutrients the body needs to function. Plasma also carries many complicated proteins that are involved in blood clotting and that help the body fight infections.

The three types of blood cells are called red cells, white cells, and platelets. The primary function of the red blood cells is to carry oxygen from the lungs to all parts of the body. They contain hemoglobin, which is the iron-containing material that gives the blood its red color and gives the cells their ability to carry oxygen. People are said to be anemic either when they do not have enough red blood cells or if the cells don't contain enough hemoglobin for some reason.

One of the most important functions of white blood cells is fighting infections. When you get a bacterial infection, the white cells go to the site of the infection and battle the bacteria by engulfing and destroying them. If you develop a bacterial infection anywhere in your body, the body immediately starts manufacturing more white blood cells to help fight the infection. The number of white cells in the blood goes up, and this fact helps doctors determine whether or not you have an internal infection and, to some extent, how serious the infection is. An infected appendix, for example, can send the white blood cell count soaring. The white cell count may also rise in certain serious conditions such as leukemia (derived from the Greek words *leukos* = white, and *haima* = blood).

The third type of cells in the blood are the platelets. These very small cells, in combination with a number of liquid proteins that are present in the plasma, are needed to form blood clots. Despite the bad reputation attributed to clotting in heart disease and stroke, the ability of the blood to clot is extremely important in maintaining the integrity of the circulatory system when even minor trauma occurs.

Even in minor accidents small blood vessels can easily become cut or torn and the blood will leak out into surrounding tissues. Unless this leakage is stopped, so much blood may be lost that the affected person may become weak or even die. The ability of the blood to clot prevents all this. As soon as a blood vessel is torn or cut, the blood-clotting system goes to work and plugs the hole with a clot. The damaged vessel then heals, and many times the affected person never even notices that much of anything has happened.

The only time blood clots are associated with illness is when the blood-clotting chain is set off by a rough spot or abnormality inside a vein that breaks off and finds its way to an important organ, plugging one of the blood vessels there that feeds the organ and compromising the organ's functioning.

Hematology and Anemia

On a visit to the doctor for a regular checkup, or if you have come with some complaint, he or she may order a complete blood count (CBC) and a study of the makeup of the plasma, often referred to as blood chemistry. A count of red blood cells checks for anemia; a count of white blood cells can help tell if an infection is caused by a bacterium or a virus; and information can be gathered about the levels of certain nutrients in the body.

Much can also be learned from analyzing the blood plasma. It can tell if there is enough water in the body, if there is something amiss with the kidneys, if there is more calcium present in the body than there should be, if your liver seems to be functioning satisfactorily, and a vast number of other things.

Anemia is a condition in which not enough oxygen is being carried to the body cells because fewer red blood cells are circulating in the bloodstream than are needed or there is less hemoglobin in the red cells than is needed. Hemoglobin is the oxygen-carrying element within the red blood cells.

Signs of anemia include pallor (sometimes noticed because the whites of the eyes are tinged with blue), pale gums, pale fingernails, fatigue, weakness, and sometimes difficulty breathing or breathlessness, even in the absence of physical exertion. When anemia is discovered, the next step is to find out what is causing it. It can be anything from undetected bleeding somewhere in the body to a vitamin deficiency or the inability of the body to absorb necessary vitamins. Vitamin B_{12} and an iron-rich diet are frequently prescribed for anemia, or if there is bleeding somewhere in the body, steps are taken to stop it.

Sickle-cell anemia is an inherited trait that attacks people of African descent almost exclusively. While there are many carriers of the gene that causes sickle-cell, fortunately only about 3 percent of the carriers actually suffer from the disease. In sickle-cell anemia, the normally round red blood cells collapse into sickle shapes which makes it harder for them to circulate in the bloodstream; capillaries may become clogged, which deprives vital organs of needed oxygen.

While a search is under way for a cure for sickle-cell anemia, there is none at present. The only prevention is in not passing the sickle-cell gene to children. If only one parent carries the sickle-cell gene, children born to these parents have a fifty-fifty chance of carrying the gene but none of them will develop the disease. If both parents carry the gene, chances are that half of their children will have the gene, and chances are that half of these will be normal and half will develop the disease. So genetic screening and counseling before they have children is desirable for couples who think they may carry the gene.

A self-test available for anemia costs about $4 in the drugstore or medical-supply store, and a more expensive test for sickle-cell anemia is about $35.

Cholesterol

Cholesterol is a substance found in all the body tissues and fluids and is used by them to produce still other substances that are essential to a variety of body functions and life itself. The body could not live without cholesterol. We get some cholesterol from foods we eat, but most of it is produced by the liver and other cells in the body. Cholesterol is carried in the bloodstream surrounded by protein shells called lipoproteins. The majority of lipoproteins in the bloodstream are low-density lipoproteins (known familiarly as LDLs), which carry the cholesterol to the cells that need it to reproduce themselves and to make hormones. There are fewer high-density lipoproteins (HDLs), which carry cholesterol back to the liver, thus lowering the total cholesterol levels in body tissues.

In some complicated way, excess LDL in the bloodstream results in deposits of cholesterol on the walls of the arteries, especially if the cholesterol it carries has been damaged by toxic products called oxidants that have been generated in the normal course of body-cell activities. Because excess LDL tends to promote the formation of fatty deposits on the walls of arteries, it has come to be known as the "bad" cholesterol, really a misnomer because, as we have seen, LDL is essential for carrying cholesterol to where it is needed and used in the process of sustaining life. On the other hand, HDL has come to be known as the "good" cholesterol because it carries away excess cholesterol and can reduce fatty deposits in the arteries.

When cholesterol first came on the public stage as being implicated in atherosclerosis, heart attack, and stroke, everyone was concerned about their "cholesterol level." A *total* cholesterol level above 200 milligrams per deciliter (200 mg/dl) was thought to put you at greater risk of arterial disease and a level below 200 indicated you were at a normal or lower risk. It soon became apparent, however, that many people with low cholesterol levels still had clogged arteries and some people with relatively high cholesterol levels had perfectly fine arteries.

Although a total cholesterol level above 200 is still looked at as risky, what is now also considered is the *ratio* of total cholesterol to HDL, the "good" cholesterol that helps limit the amount of fatty deposits on artery walls. This is expressed as total cholesterol ÷ HDL cholesterol.

Cholesterol Testing

At this writing, kits to self-test for total cholesterol level are available at the drugstore.
You have to follow the instructions on the
package very carefully to obtain an accurate
result. These kits can tell you if your total
cholesterol level is considered acceptable or
higher than might be good for you, but they
do not provide the essential information
about the total cholesterol to HDL cholesterol ratio. Newer kits may do this in the
future, but at the moment the test still has
to be done through your doctor.

The cholesterol test by a hospital laboratory or in your doctor's office consists of taking a blood sample first thing in the morning
before you have had anything to eat or drink.
Doctors usually request that you fast for at
least fifteen hours before a blood sample is
taken for the results of your test to be accurate. When you get the results, ask your doctor what your total cholesterol is and what the
HDL cholesterol is. Then divide the total cholesterol by the HDL cholesterol. Examples:

- Total cholesterol is 190 mg/dl and
  HDL cholesterol is 30 mg/dl

  $$190 \div 30 = 6.3:1$$

- Total cholesterol is 230 mg/dl and
  HDL is 50 mg/dl

  $$230 \div 50 = 4.6:1$$

Currently, five is considered a bench-
mark for what is considered a "desirable"
cholesterol ratio. In recent studies a ratio of
four seemed to reduce a person's risk of
heart attack by more than 50 percent.

In the first example, the ratio of 6.3 is
considered high. In the second example,
although the total cholesterol is relatively
high, the ratio of 4.6 seems to put the patient
at lower risk of heart attack than the general
population, according to current thinking.

Exercise seems to be a good way to
increase your HDL level. There are ongoing
studies about the effects of diet on HDL and
LDL, but there is little that can be said with
certainty at the moment. Obesity, on the
other hand, seems to be clearly related to
high levels of LDL, the "bad" cholesterol. So
the best advice for keeping your cholesterol
ratios where they should be is still exercise,
a sensible low-fat diet, and weight reduction.

The Circulatory System

The blood, pumped by the heart, circulates
through the body in a branching system of
arteries and veins. It is the arteries that carry
newly oxygenated blood from the heart,
beginning with a single major artery called the
aorta, which branches into smaller and smaller
arteries until the branches are so small they
can't be seen with the naked eye. These smallest branches are called capillaries, which are
very thin-walled vessels that can keep the
blood cells in circulation but allow oxygen,
nutrients, and other chemical substances to
pass through to feed body tissues and allow
carbon dioxide and other waste products to be
picked up by the blood and carried away to be
disposed of. The capillaries then lead into
larger and larger vessels, the veins, until they
all join in a single large vessel called the vena
cava, which returns the blood to the heart.

When you cut yourself superficially, the bleeding is from capillaries and small veins. In more deeply penetrating wounds, a larger vein or even a small artery may be cut, and the bleeding is more severe. Blood from veins and capillaries tends to ooze and dribble out of a cut, while arterial blood, which is under much higher pressure, may actually come out in squirts each time the heart beats. Even small arteries may spurt blood a foot or more out of the wound.

How to Deal with Bleeding

1. Even small wounds may be frightening because the blood quickly runs and spreads, making a mess. Find the source of the bleeding and determine if the blood is oozing or spurting from the wound.

2. The first line of defense in any bleeding is applying pressure to the wound with a pad of sterile gauze. Lacking this, use the cleanest thing available—a clean handkerchief, washcloth, sanitary napkin, etc. If blood is spurting, indicating that an artery has been cut, get emergency help at once and maintain pressure on the wound while you are waiting for the ambulance.

3. Elevating the wound above the level of the heart will help slow bleeding. Do not elevate an arm or leg, however, if you also suspect a bone may have been broken.

4. Even severe cuts will tend to be stopped by the clotting process if continuous pressure is maintained over the wound from ten to twenty minutes. If blood soaks through the pad you have placed over the wound, don't remove it for this may interfere with the clotting that is taking place. Apply a new bandage over the old one and continue to apply pressure. If you can't continue to hold the cover over the wound, wrap a bandage tightly around it to maintain the pressure.

5. If there is severe arterial bleeding from a wound in an arm or leg that you are unable to stop by applying pressure over the wound and you are a long way from emergency medical help, you can try to slow the bleeding at pressure points where a major artery crosses a bone. There is a pressure point inside the arm just below the armpit where the major artery to the arm crosses the bone of the upper arm. By grasping the arm and applying pressure with your fingers at this point, you may be able to slow or stop the bleeding. A pressure point for the leg is located in the middle of the crease that the front of your leg makes where it joins the torso. Apply pressure at this point with the heel of your hand. Pressure directly over the wound should be maintained at the same time.

Aneurysms in Blood Vessels

Arteries and veins, because of the difference in the thickness of their walls and the difference of the blood pressure inside them, develop different kinds of problems. Two of the most important problems that arteries may fall heir to, especially as we get older and there is atherosclerosis (hardening of the arteries), are the development of aneurysms and blockages.

Aneurysms are ball-like swellings that happen when the wall of an artery becomes weakened. Any artery can develop an aneurysm, but they are most common in the brain and in the aorta, the big artery that runs through the chest and abdomen down to the legs. If there is a weak spot in the wall of an artery, it may begin to swell (much like the wall of a tire or inner tube does when it has been weakened), and as the swelling gets larger the vessel wall becomes even weaker. Eventually, the aneurysm may break, leaking blood into surrounding tissues. In both the brain and the aorta, this is an extremely serious event, and in both cases the affected person may die even if the condition is quickly recognized and appropriate action is taken.

Aneurysms of the brain are generally found with magnetic resonance imaging (MRI), but this test is used only when a problem is suspected for some reason, not for general screening. An aneurysm in the aorta may be discovered, however, in a chest x-ray—one reason that doctors recommend a chest x-ray every few years in older people. An aneurysm farther down the aorta, in the abdomen, can also be discovered in an x-ray, or it may be felt in the course of palpating the abdomen (pressing firmly into the abdomen and feeling with the fingers), something a doctor always does in a general physical exam for this and a number of other reasons we will discuss in other chapters.

Feeling for an Aortic Aneurysm in the Abdomen

1. The person being examined should be flat on his or her back and asked to relax the abdomen as much as possible. It will be easier to do this examination with a thin person and quite difficult if there is a lot of abdominal fat to feel through.

2. Palpate (feel) in the center line of the abdomen, working your way down from just below the breastbone to the pelvic area. You palpate by placing the flats of the fingers of your left hand on your abdomen. Press down with your right hand on the fingers of the left hand. Your right hand should apply the pressure while the fingers of your left hand do the feeling.

3. An aneurysm will feel like a round mass, perhaps the size of a small orange, that is pulsating regularly as the heart beats. In very thin people, a normal aorta may feel like a pulsating tubelike structure. This is perfectly normal. But if you can feel a pulsating ball-like mass, an aneurysm may be developing and you should seek medical attention promptly. Aneurysms can be treated successfully if they are caught before they begin to crack or leak.

Blockages in Arteries

Arteries can also develop blockages. Blockages occur most often because of the buildup of cholesterol and related substances on the internal walls of the arteries and can happen at almost any place in the arterial system. This is a very slow process and there is good evidence now that, by lowering cholesterol and other blood-fat components, the fatty buildup can actually be reversed. This may be accomplished through changes in diet and changes in lifestyle and by medication if necessary.

The most well known of arterial blockages is, of course, the heart attack. Heart attacks occur when blood vessels feeding some part of the heart muscle become blocked, leaving the muscle unable to function because it has lost its blood supply. Angina and heart attack were discussed in Chapter 1. When an artery in the brain or leading to the brain becomes blocked, the result is a stroke.

Two carotid arteries branch off of the aorta (the main artery leading out of the heart) and pass through the neck on their way to the brain. One artery supplies one side of the brain and the other artery provides blood for the other half. You can make a basic evaluation of these two vital arteries yourself with a few simple observations and the use of your stethoscope.

Examining the Carotid Arteries

1. The first step in your evaluation of the carotid arteries consists of visual observation. The two carotid arteries enter the neck behind the two bony prominences at the base of the neck commonly known as the collarbones. Carefully observe this area of the neck. Except during vigorous physical exer-

tion or extreme emotional distress, you should not be able to detect with your eyes the pulsation of the carotid arteries. These arteries may throb visibly, however, in aged people and in those suffering from high blood pressure, hyperthyroidism, and anemia. If you are able to see the pulsation of the carotid arteries in your neck, you should bring this finding to the attention of your doctor.

2. Now locate the pulse points of the carotid arteries. To do this, place your fingertips at the angle of your jaw just below the earlobes; now bring them down an inch or two and you should be able to feel the pulsation of the carotid arteries. Do not press too hard or too long on a carotid artery. First feel one carotid pulse and then the other, and compare the strength of the two. They should be approximately equal. A carotid pulse that seems markedly weaker than the other may indicate a narrowing of that carotid artery. This is an important finding that your doctor should know about.

3. Finally, take your stethoscope and listen to the carotid arteries. Following the instructions for the use of the stethoscope given in Chapter 1, place the chest piece on the carotid pulse. Be sure to hold your breath while you listen or you will hear great, loud rushes of air each time you take a breath.

4. Normally, you should hear nothing at all when you listen to the carotid pulse using

a stethoscope; if anything, you may hear your heart beating faintly in the distance. Should there be an area of constriction somewhere along the artery, however, the flow of blood through the vessel will make a whooshing sound. Doctors call this a *bruit*, which is simply French for "noise." If you think you hear this whooshing sound and you are sure it's not just the sound of your breathing, you should have your suspicions checked out by a doctor.

Signs and Symptoms of Stroke

While some of the following symptoms may indicate problems other than a stroke, they should still be cause to seek immediate medical attention:

- Unexplained dizziness, confusion, or unsteadiness

- A change in mental ability; loss of ability to concentrate

- Decreased consciousness

- Loss of vision, double vision, or dimness, particularly in one eye

- Weakness, numbness, or paralysis of arms, legs, or face, often on just one side

- Inability to speak or trouble speaking

- Sudden severe headache that is different from other headaches normally experienced

Arteries in the arms and legs may also experience blockages, though the legs are the more common sites for this to happen. The affected limb will develop a blanched, white look and will become weaker and weaker because it has lost its blood supply. This is a medical emergency. If treatment is not begun soon, the affected limb may gradually start to die and will have to be amputated.

Signs of a Blocked Artery in a Limb

1. Compare the affected limb with its opposite. With an arterial blockage, the affected limb will look whiter.

2. If an arm is affected, check for a pulse at the wrist. If a leg is affected, check for a pulse at the ankle or on top of the foot. You will not be able to feel a pulse if there is a blockage.

Blockages in Veins

Veins have thinner walls than arteries do, and the pressure inside veins is much lower; consequently, veins develop different kinds of problems. Two important and well-known problems that occur in veins are thrombophlebitis, or simply phlebitis, and varicose veins. (The imposing sixteen-letter word, thrombophlebitis, breaks down into Greek-originating parts that pretty well describe what is going on. *Thrombos* is a clot; *phleps* is a blood vessel; and an *itis* is a disease or inflammation.)

Phlebitis occurs most commonly in the legs. It often begins after a long period of inactivity, such as when a person is confined to bed or has been sitting for a long time, especially in a seat with a prominent edge that tends to press on the veins. An historical case of phlebitis occurred when President Richard Nixon suffered this ailment during a transatlantic flight.

Venous blood flow, particularly in the legs, depends in part on the activity of the leg muscles around the veins. As the muscles move they put pressure on the veins with a pumping action that helps move the blood along. When there is little movement of the muscles, the blood flow may become very sluggish, and a clot may form, especially if rough spots caused by minor damage or aging are inside the vein .

A blood clot in a vein is a condition that should not be ignored, because if it is not properly treated it can break off and lodge in another part of the body. The most serious event is a clot that goes through the heart and out into the lungs, obstructs blood flow to the lungs, and severely limits the ability to breathe. This is called a pulmonary embolism and is a medical emergency.

When to Suspect Phlebitis

1. There is unexplained pain in one leg, frequently in the calf.

2. There may be swelling, with the leg feeling heavy and sensitive to touch.

3. Take the affected calf in both hands and squeeze it gently. Do the same with the unaffected calf. The affected calf should be more tender.

4. Measure both calves with a tape measure. Move the tape measure up and down a bit to make sure you are measuring the fattest part of the calf. If the calf on the affected side is a quarter inch or more larger than the other side, you should be concerned and see a doctor as soon as possible.

Varicose Veins

Varicose veins occur when the surface veins of the legs become enlarged and swollen and show blue through the skin. Varicose veins tend to get worse rather than better as time goes by, and some blood clots may form in them, but they do not tend to break off or cause serious problems elsewhere. Varicose veins swell and become evident as blue, bulging veins when you are standing and will subside by emptying themselves when you lie down with your legs elevated slightly above the level of the heart. But, unfortunately, the veins will refill and bulge again when you stand.

Doctors generally recommend wearing elastic stockings if you have varicose veins to keep some pressure on the legs and flatten out the veins. This will not cure varicose veins but will help prevent the veins from stretching further. The only cure for varicose veins is a surgical operation known as vein stripping.

The Lymph System

Lymph is a plasmalike substance that drains from body tissues in a system of vessels called lymph vessels, or lymphatics. The lymph flowing through these vessels eventually empties into the bloodstream via a large vein in the neck. Lymph nodes, tiny beanlike structures, are clustered along the lymph vessels. These nodes capture infecting organisms or foreign particles that get into the body from disease, injury, or in other ways. The nodes then become major sites for battles between the invaders and protective scavenger cells of the body.

The body has a large number of lymph nodes located in the neck, behind the ears, in the armpits, behind and above the elbows, in the area of the groin, and in the hollow of each collarbone. Most of the time these nodes are too small to be seen or felt. Enlarged lymph nodes are a sure sign that the body is fighting off an infection of some kind. As a node accumulates more and more material, it enlarges and you can feel it quite readily.

Nodes in the neck and the jaw area commonly swell as a reaction to a toothache, sores in the mouth, or a viral respiratory infection such as the flu. Swollen nodes behind the ears suggest German measles, a sore on the scalp, or an ear infection, while enlarged nodes in front of the ears point to some problem in the area of the face and eyes. Nodes in the armpits may swell in response to injuries and subsequent infections in the arms or hands, while swollen nodes in the groin may appear with some injury to the legs or feet.

Finally, all the lymph nodes in your body may be swollen in response to a generalized infection such as mononucleosis or more serious systemic diseases. Any swollen lymph nodes should be reported to the doctor so that treatment of whatever is causing the swelling can begin.

Examining the Lymph Nodes in the Neck

You are probably most familiar with the doctor feeling for swollen lymph nodes in your neck when you have a cold, sore throat, or earache; that examination is described here. Feeling for swollen lymph nodes in the armpits and groin follows the same procedure.

1. With your fingers together, use the fleshy pads of the fingers to feel for lymph nodes along the entire course of the neck. Try to relax your neck muscles while you do this. Make sure your examination extends around to the back of the neck, up under the chin, and at the angle of the jaw as well.

2. A swollen lymph node may feel soft or hard and may or may not be painful when you press on it. But usually a node that has enlarged because of a simple infection feels soft and is painful when you poke at it.

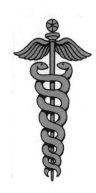

3

How to Examine and Test Your Digestive System

The digestive tract gets more media time than any other part of the body, and for people who manufacture things for the "tummy" and other parts of the alimentary canal, it's money well spent. The return in sales of laxatives, antacids, and other over-the-counter drugs for the gastrointestinal tract is a multibillion-dollar industry. Still, most people know surprisingly little about this remarkable machinery that rumbles and grumbles while it does its essential job of feeding the body.

The best way to get acquainted with your digestive organs is through a laying on of hands, called palpating, probing and pushing into your abdomen as your doctor does in the course of an examination. Under normal circumstances there's not much to feel except muscle and fat and an occasional slippery thing sliding under your fingers, which is exactly what the doctor feels when he or she presses and probes. But it's a good way to remember where everything is, and it's

important to know what your abdomen feels like when it's well so that you have a basis for comparison when you suspect something may be wrong.

Locating the Organs of the Digestive System

Except for the mouth and the esophagus—the tube leading from the mouth to the stomach—all the organs involved in digestion are located in the abdominal cavity, the lower part of the torso below the diaphragm. The diaphragm is the dome-shaped muscular partition that separates the organs of the chest cavity—the heart and lungs—from those in the abdominal cavity.

Six organs in the abdominal cavity work in the digestive process: the stomach, the liver, the gallbladder, the pancreas, and about thirty feet of small and large intestines. This digestive machinery shares the

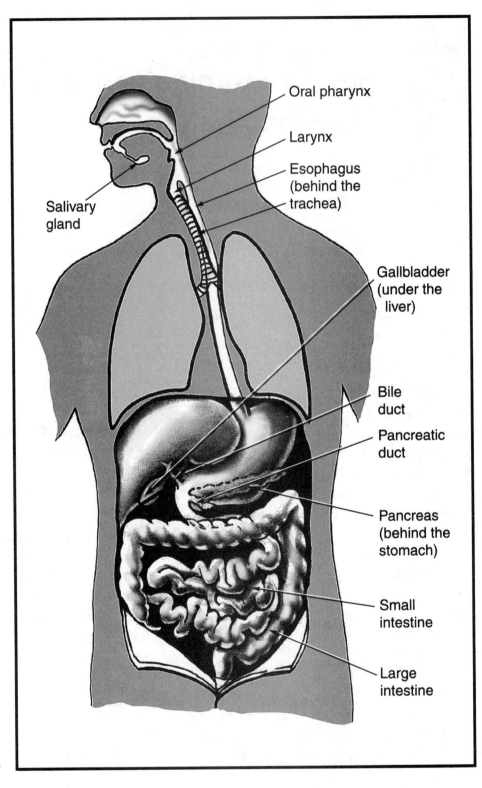

*Organs of the
Digestive System*

abdomen with the spleen, kidneys, urinary bladder, and the reproductive organs in women, which makes for a somewhat crowded neighborhood, but each organ has its place and, generally speaking, they get along well together.

General Instructions for Palpating the Abdomen

You can feel your own abdomen or work with a partner. The directions locate organs on *your own* right or left side. If you work with a partner, therefore, keep in mind where your partner's left and right sides are as you face one another.

1. Draw two imaginary lines through your navel—one vertically and one horizontally—to divide your abdomen into four quadrants. Lie comfortably on your back and relax your abdomen.

2. Place the flats of the fingers of your left hand on your abdomen. Press down on top of your left fingers with your right hand. Your right hand should apply the pressure while your left fingers do the feeling.

3. You can exert a good bit of pressure as you feel about, but use good sense. Your object is not to see if you can hurt yourself. If you intend to work with a partner, practice on yourself first, then make allowances for the size of your partner. You want to use much less pres-

sure on a child than on a large, heavily muscled man.

The Liver and the Gallbladder

The liver is a very large organ, much larger than most people think, and it has many functions in maintaining and monitoring body chemistry. One of its important functions is to produce bile, a chemical agent that helps break down fats so that they can be digested. Bile is pumped from the liver into the small intestine via the gallbladder, a small organ shaped like a tiny eggplant that hangs below the liver. Bile is stored in the gallbladder in concentrated form until it is needed. When fats enter the small intestine, the gallbladder contracts and squirts out some bile. But bile can also go directly from the liver to the intestine, which is why you can get along very nicely without a gallbladder when it must be removed.

Locating the Liver and Gallbladder

1. Find the gristly bottom tip of your breastbone that feels like a little lump just before you get into the soft, fleshy part of the abdomen. This is called the xiphoid (zy'-foid) process, a bump that sometimes alarms people the first time they find it because they think it is some sort of tumor. You are now on the vertical midline that you drew through the navel. The diaphragm is just above this point, so you are at the upper limit of the abdomen. Part of your liver is directly underneath.

2. From the xiphoid process, run your fingers down diagonally to the right along the bottom of the right rib cage. When you reach the bottom of your rib cage, where the last rib turns toward your back, you have finally reached the lower right limits of your liver. It is a huge organ, the largest in your body. The rest lies tucked up under your right rib cage and its top rests against the diaphragm.

3. Go back to a point along the bottom of the rib cage that is about on a line drawn down from your right nipple. You are now in the vicinity of where the gallbladder is hanging under the liver. You will not feel it unless it is giving you distress.

4. Lay the flats of the fingers of your left hand on your abdomen at this point with the index finger just rubbing against the rib cage. Apply pressure with your right hand on top of the left fingers.

5. Now let the air out of your lungs, press down with your hand, and take a deep breath. As you breathe in, you may feel the edge of your liver pass under the fingers of your left hand either right under the rib cage or two to three finger widths below it. Whether or not you feel your liver depends on how you are built and how perceptive you are with your hands. But the real purpose of this examination is to get the hang of feeling your abdomen and to learn where your liver and gallbladder are.

The Stomach and the Esophagus

The tough, cartilaginous tube that you can feel in the front part of your neck is the trachea, or windpipe, which carries air to the lungs. The esophagus, a muscular tube that carries food from the mouth to the stomach, is located directly behind the trachea and in front of the vertebrae in your neck, so it's quite inaccessible for feeling. The only time you become aware of the esophagus is when something very cold, very hot, or very lumpy seems to take its time traveling down into the stomach.

The esophagus is ten to twelve inches long in most adults and most of that length is in the throat and the chest. The esophagus pierces the diaphragm at about the level of the xiphoid process and makes a gentle turn to the left for about an inch and enters the stomach. Stomachs have roughly a J shape, but they can't be depended on to have precisely the same shape and location in everyone, so the following description may not be exactly right for you, though it is probably close.

Locating the Stomach

Contrary to common belief and erroneous diagrams shown on television antacid commercials, the bulk of most stomachs lies just slightly left of center in the abdomen. Usually, not much more than a quarter of the stomach crosses the midline to the right where it meets the small intestine.

1. Place your fingers on the xiphoid process. This is about where the esophagus enters the stomach.

2. Draw a line from the xiphoid process on a slight downward slope to a point on your left rib cage that is about two inches below your left nipple. This is the approximate location of the left limit of your stomach, which means that part of the stomach, like the liver, is nestled up under the dome-shaped diaphragm and is partially protected by the rib cage.

3. Drop down a bit and circle to the right across your abdomen almost, but not quite, to the point on your right rib cage where you poked about for your liver. This is the right lower limit of the stomach in most people, where it joins the small intestine. And both stomach and small intestine may be under the bottom edge of the liver at this point.

4. If you push in with your fingers after a large meal, you should feel more fullness discomfort in the area described than you will by pushing into the abdomen lower down, around the navel, or below, for example. Keep in mind, however, that a few very normal stomachs do descend as low as the navel or further. What we have described are "average" stomachs.

Go back to the left rib cage for a moment, just under the left nipple. The spleen is tucked up in here between the stomach and the left side of the left rib cage. The spleen is not related to the digestive tract. It is a filter and storage center for blood cells. Once again, while palpating around the stomach area and then under the left rib cage, you are not likely to feel anything but soft, fleshy tissue. With some blood diseases or infections, the spleen may become enlarged, in which case the tip of it may be felt around the left rib cage.

The Small Intestine

Most of the abdominal cavity is filled with the small intestine. This mass of tubing, between twenty and thirty feet of it, begins at the bottom right end of the stomach and winds around and around until it ends in the large intestine on the lower right side of the abdomen. The reason for its great length is that most digestion and absorption of food takes place here, and a great deal of surface area is required.

Draw a line across the bottom edges of the rib cages, then go down to the pelvis on each side, and then across to the top of the urinary bladder—where the feeling of fullness is when you have to urinate. All of the area within these boundaries is filled with the small intestine. Pressing into this area should reveal no hard spots or any discomfort aside from what you would normally expect from being poked.

Tracing the Large Intestine

The large intestine—called the colon—is the last part of the digestive tract. The residue of undigested food accumulates here and is made ready for evacuation by a bit more absorption of nutrients and the removal of water. The colon forms a sort of picture frame around the small intestine.

1. Find a spot on the vertical midline of the abdomen about halfway between the navel and the top of the urinary bladder. Now draw your fingers to the right until you meet the pelvis. The beginning of the large intestine is just about here, sitting in the inside hollow of the right pelvic bone.

2. Probe around a bit just under the edge of the bone and consider what goes on here. The small intestine is joined to the large intestine at this point. The large intestine—the colon—rises from this point to the bottom of the liver, and so this section is called the ascending colon. But there is also a small section of colon, called the cecum, that goes down an inch or so to a dead end. The appendix is attached to the cecum like a large, dangling worm that can be anywhere from two to six inches long. It extends inward, to the left a bit, from the cecum, and this is the site of appendicitis when it strikes.

3. Draw a line upward to where you felt for your liver. The ascending colon makes a right-angle turn here and goes to about the same site under the left rib cage. This section is called the transverse colon because it goes across.

4. Another right-angle turn takes the descending colon down to about the center of the left pelvis where it makes

another sharp turn and goes a bit inward—this is now the sigmoid colon, which travels a short way to the rectum and so to the outside world.

Other Organs of the Abdomen

The pancreas is the only other organ in the abdomen that is directly associated with the digestive process. It is buried deep in the abdomen, well hidden by the stomach and small intestine, and is even difficult to show in a diagram. One of its functions is to produce a group of important digestive enzymes that, like bile, are pumped into the small intestine. Its other important function is to produce insulin, which controls blood sugar. The body's failure to control blood sugar, resulting in diabetes, will be discussed in Chapter 11, which deals with metabolic disorders.

The pancreas has a long tail that runs from the spleen in the upper left quadrant, under the stomach, and ends in a head that is tucked under one of the curves of the small intestine in the vicinity of the right rib cage. Because it is so inaccessible, trouble here is very hard to detect.

The kidneys, urinary bladder, ovaries, and uterus—all discussed in other parts of this book—complete the roll call of abdominal organs.

After you have explored your own and one or two other abdomens, you should have a pretty good idea of what an abdomen feels like and about where everything is. Probe every six months or so and in times of abdominal distress. If you feel pain or hard spots or lumpy matter anywhere, it should be reported to a doctor. Be sure, of course, that you don't create pain with overly zealous probing. Have warm hands and probe deliberately. A light touch tickles. Remember, you will always find one little lump in the middle of the abdomen at the end of the breastbone—the xiphoid process, which countless people fear is an abnormal growth when they first discover it.

The Digestion Process

The first step in the digestion process is chewing. Chewing is important because it breaks food into small particles that then can be worked on by the various chemicals in the mouth, the stomach, and the small intestine. As you chew, saliva pours into the mouth from two little pimplelike outlets that are approximately in the center of your cheeks and can be seen rather easily in a simple inspection of the mouth, using a flashlight. Saliva wets down food, making it easier to swallow, and begins the digestive process by turning some starches into sugar.

Sometimes, when certain kinds of foods—corn, for example—are not well chewed, they go right through the entire intestinal tract without being digested and are evacuated in the stools in almost the same condition as when they were eaten. Thorough chewing has many salutary effects: It aids digestion, it can help reduce indigestion, it helps in weight-loss programs because you feel full and satisfied sooner, and it can help reduce problems with gas—all good reasons why your mother

was right when she said, "Eat slowly, chew well, and don't talk with a full mouth."

When food is swallowed, it moves to the stomach through the esophagus. Where the esophagus joins the stomach is a circular muscle, the cardiac sphincter, that opens to let food into the stomach and then closes to keep it there. Beginning with the esophagus, food is moved along the entire alimentary canal (the digestive tract) by a series of wavelike contractions in the walls of the tubing. This is called peristalsis and it moves food in about the same way that you squeeze toothpaste through a tube.

Once in the stomach, food is treated with acid to break it up further and with enzymes that help prepare some of the nutrients for absorption in the small intestine. Some water, certain drugs, and alcohol are absorbed in the stomach, but this is not its primary function.

When food is liquid enough or the pieces are small enough, they are squirted from the stomach into the small intestine through the pyloric sphincter, another muscular gatekeeper. The small intestine consists of three sections—the duodenum, the jejunum, and the ileum—although there is no really perceptible dividing point between one section and another.

At the beginning of the small intestine, the duodenum, bile is introduced from the liver via the gallbladder and a bile duct, enzymes arrive from the pancreas via the pancreatic duct, and other enzymes are produced by cells of the intestine. All of this chemical processing changes the composition of food to a form that can be absorbed and used by the body.

Food absorption requires a large surface, which is why the small intestine is so long. In addition, the walls of the intestine are lined with millions of finger-shaped projections called villi, which are so small that they are just barely visible to the unaided eye. These add tremendously to the absorption surface of the intestine. The villi are rich in capillaries—tiny blood vessels—and prepared nutrients from the intestine pass into them. Larger blood vessels then carry the nutrients to the liver, where they are sorted and processed further before going on to the rest of the body.

You will recall that the parts of the colon are the cecum—the dead-end section at the beginning with the appendix attached to it—the ascending colon, the transverse colon, the descending colon, the sigmoid colon, and the rectum.

There is yet another valve where the small intestine joins the large intestine that admits the residue of undigested food into the colon but allows nothing to flow back. A little bit more food value is extracted in the colon, but mostly water is absorbed there and the remaining material is compacted, mixed with a large number of bacteria, and prepared for elimination.

Friendly bacteria that inhabit the colon perform vital functions such as producing some vitamins, fermenting undigested food, and combating harmful bacteria that may have been introduced into the colon. When under abnormal circumstances these friendly bacteria are killed off (during treatment with superpotent antibiotics, for example), diarrhea, cramps, and even intestinal bleeding may occur until the normal bacterial population can be restored.

Food residue is quite watery as it enters the ascending colon, but by the time it reaches the sigmoid colon it is fairly firm and compact—the very familiar feces. If it becomes too dry, constipation may result; not dry enough and you may have symptoms of diarrhea. Once or twice a day, or less frequently in some people, the compacted residue moves into the rectum where nerve endings signal a feeling of fullness. When you voluntarily relax the anal sphincter at the end of the rectum, the fecal material passes to the outside world.

Looking at and Listening to Your Abdomen

Get to know what your abdomen looks like. If your body is changing, all the doctor can see is what it looks like at the moment of the examination. It's helpful to know what your body was like before and how fast the change is occurring. If you have become paunchy, has the paunchiness occurred high, or low, or all over? What were your measurements six months ago, a year ago? Paunchiness may be the result of simple weight gain or loss of muscle tone (which is bad enough), but it can also result from organ enlargement or the accumulation of fluid, either condition being cause for serious concern. Isolated lumps, bumps, and swellings should always be viewed with suspicion, of course, and called to a doctor's attention.

An interesting way to check the general level of function of your intestinal tract is to listen to your abdomen with your stethoscope.

1. Place the stethoscope in your ears the same way you did when listening to your heart. Place the end of the stethoscope over various areas of your abdomen.

2. You will hear a type of gurgling sound that is not at all constant. Sometimes you hear nothing at all for a period of ten to fifteen seconds, followed by a series of gurgles that last perhaps five seconds. The sound of the gurgles varies from a sort of low-pitched groan to a medium-pitched sloshing sound. These sounds differ slightly from one area of the abdomen to another.

3. Listen to various parts of your abdomen when you are feeling well and become familiar with normal gurgling. Try it just before, just after, and between meals, because sounds will also vary depending on the extent of activity going on.

4. If a bowel obstruction occurs, the sounds change markedly. After a few hours all normal bowel sounds disappear. The abdomen becomes quiet except for high-pitched tinkling sounds. Or the sounds are sometimes described as water slowly dripping inside a sewer pipe—high-pitched and ringing in nature. Although the sounds are neither loud nor dramatic, they are very important and indicate the need for immediate medical treatment.

Distress, Bleeding, and Other Symptoms in the Digestive System

When something goes wrong with the digestive system and related organs it will become manifest in a number of ways: pain, nausea, vomiting, diarrhea, weakness, dizziness, and sweating. Bleeding can occur at any point within the digestive tract and may or may not be noticed easily. When the liver and gallbladder are involved in a disorder, yellowing (jaundice) can appear in the skin or the whites of the eyes. Blurring of vision, muscle weakness, and other signs that the nervous system has been affected may occur in cases of serious food poisoning.

Digestive upsets are so common and familiar that most people hate to make a fuss over an "upset stomach" or "a little indigestion" until the distress really becomes severe and no longer can be ignored. It is not at all easy to know when to worry about digestive upset or abdominal pain. But if you are familiar with the normal feel of your abdomen, if you know where the organs are located, and if you have become used to tracking the functioning of your body with a high degree of awareness, the decision making can be done more intelligently. Here are some tips for tracking and observation.

Occasional Distress Versus Severe Pain

It is entirely possible to experience quite uncomfortable abdominal pain that is of no serious medical consequence. This pain is usually of rather short duration and may be quite severe for a few minutes, disappear completely for a while, and then come back again. Persistent discomfort of this type should, however, be investigated.

Do not ignore stabbing or piercing acute pain or continuous pain of increasing intensity. Even a steady, dull ache can be significant if it is continuous. This kind of pain should be looked into by a physician without delay. In years gone by, it would be said that someone died of "acute indigestion," when it was really a heart attack and the pain was mistaken for a stomachache.

Indigestion Versus Heart Pain

Indigestion is a catchall, imprecise term for a wide variety of symptoms including different kinds of pain, nausea, heartburn, and gas. It may be occasional and temporary, brought on by some type of overindulgence or stress, or it may indicate something more serious. One clue is frequency of recurrence and the persistence of the distress. Track symptoms carefully: time and circumstances of onset, duration, suspect food eaten or drugs taken (including coffee, tobacco, and alcohol), and the precise location and nature of the distress. Then, if you have to report to a physician, you can do it accurately and intelligently.

Pain high up in the abdomen is usually referred to as a stomachache because the stomach is located under the diaphragm,

right at the base of the breastbone. It is indeed here that the pain from a peptic ulcer, a hiatus hernia, or even just a plain old green-apples tummyache occurs. It is important to know, however, that it is not always possible to distinguish pain in this area from chest pain caused by heart problems. A rather sudden onset of pain high up in your abdomen might indicate heart disease rather than stomach problems.

A fine line exists between running to the doctor for every pain and ignoring something serious, and that's why it is important for you to know your health history, to know where things are located in your body, and to know how your body normally operates. Anything different, severe, or persistent should be investigated.

Reflux and Hiatus Hernia

Reflux simply means a flowing backward. When applied to the digestive system, it most often refers to the flowing backward of stomach contents up into the esophagus. When this highly acid material flows into the esophagus, it causes a sensation of burning and pain. It occurs more often when you are lying down than when you are upright because of the effects of gravity on the stomach contents. Backflow is normally prevented by a muscular ring called a sphincter, a type of valve found at several places throughout the intestinal tract that opens and closes at appropriate times to let intestinal contents through and prevent it from flowing back. The one at the junction of the stomach and the esophagus is called the cardiac sphincter, and when this becomes weak, reflux occurs.

One of the reasons that the cardiac sphincter may not function properly is a condition called hiatus hernia. A hiatus is simply a hole through which a structure passes, and in this case it is the hole in the diaphragm through which the esophagus passes to reach the stomach. When this hole becomes stretched or enlarged, the stomach can actually poke its way up into the chest, and this is called a hiatus hernia. The term hernia is applied whenever an organ is able to push its way through a hole that is supposed to be tight. We will encounter this term again when we talk about inguinal hernia, a condition where a section of the intestine can poke its way through the inguinal ring in the groin area.

When a piece of stomach works its way into the chest cavity and becomes a hiatus hernia, there is irritation and pain because, once again, it allows the acidic stomach contents to back up into the esophagus. And, once again, it often occurs when you are lying down because there is no pull of gravity to keep the flow of stomach contents going downward.

The pain associated with a hiatus hernia may mimic a heart attack, complete with a dull ache in the chest and radiating pain to the shoulder. The differences are that the pain of a hiatus hernia occurs most often after a meal, does not worsen with effort, and is noticed most when lying down or bending over. Standing and walking around can actually relieve the symptoms. But if you have pain that resembles a heart attack that hasn't been diagnosed before as a hiatus hernia, it is best to check it out and be sure.

Inguinal Hernia

An inguinal hernia is a bulging in the groin area caused by a section of intestine that has slipped through a passage in the inguinal ring. This passage originally allowed the testicles to move from the body where they were formed into the scrotum. The passage normally becomes sealed afterward, but if the seal is not tight, the weakness may become evident when a piece of intestine is able to push its way through the inguinal ring. The hernia often happens after lifting heavy objects. It can also happen in women, but not nearly so frequently as in men because corresponding passages in the inguinal ring are much smaller in women than in men.

In the most severe cases, a loop of intestine can go all the way down into the scrotum, which causes the scrotum to become seriously enlarged. But the more common event is for a swelling to appear on one or both sides in the groin area.

An inguinal hernia should be repaired for two reasons: First, the piece of bowel slipping through the inguinal ring may become swollen and unable to work its way back into the abdominal cavity. The blood supply may become pinched off and the bowel will become dying tissue. This requires emergency surgery. The other reason is that as time goes by the weakness becomes worse and more and more bowel is able to push its way into the scrotum.

Most hernias can be pushed back into the abdomen if you lie on your back and gently massage and press the swollen area. You will feel the loop of bowel pop back through the hole into the abdomen. This is called reducing the hernia, but it doesn't last very long; the hernia will pop out again unless it is surgically repaired.

Pain of Appendicitis

Appendicitis is very difficult to diagnose, even for a physician. If you suspect appendicitis, it should be reported to a physician at once for evaluation. Suspicious signs include:

- Pain starting near the navel that migrates to the right lower quadrant of the abdomen and settles there

- Tenderness in the right lower quadrant on deep palpation and absence of similar tenderness on the left side

- Some degree of muscle spasm on the right side (this can be felt if you are familiar with your abdomen). Similar pain on the left side, if severe and persistent, may indicate diverticular disease—pouches forming on the descending colon— and must be checked by a physician.

- Low fever—100° to 101° F or a little bit higher

Gallbladder Pain

Gallbladder pain, which can be severe and knifelike, occurs in the upper right quadrant of the abdomen. Onset of pain may be associated with a fatty meal. It may last several hours and then gradually go away. Then pain is likely to recur when another fatty meal is eaten. The pain may radiate up into the chest where it is most commonly felt in the area of the right shoulder blade. So severe knifelike pain should be investigated at once because the pain of gallbladder inflammation and heart attack can be confused, and they occur with most frequency in people who are most susceptible through age and lifestyle to both ailments.

Ulcer and Pancreas Pain

Pain from an ulcer either in the stomach (peptic ulcer) or in the small intestine (duodenal ulcer) usually occurs high and in the middle of the abdomen. It is often so well localized that you can point to the exact spot where the pain is felt. Pain from an inflammation of the pancreas also occurs high and in the middle of the abdomen. Pain from any of these sources can be quite severe, burning, or gnawing and may pierce through to the back. Ulcer pain can usually be associated with eating in the following way: Pain may appear a few hours after a meal and then is relieved when something is eaten again. Incidentally, it should be kept in mind that ulcers are not uncommon in children and young adults as well as in older people.

Hemorrhoids

Hemorrhoids consist of swollen veins in the area of the anal canal and sphincter. Hemorrhoids are classified as internal or external depending on whether they develop just inside or just outside the anal sphincter. There may be a mixture of both. They tend to hurt, itch, and bleed. Bleeding appears as bright red blood in the toilet or as spots of blood on toilet tissue. This bleeding is not dangerous and hemorrhoids do not degenerate into cancer. People with hemorrhoids often panic the first time they notice the bright red blood of bleeding in the toilet or staining their underwear. It should be checked out by your doctor the first time, but after that bleeding can easily be stopped with a clean pad.

Hemorrhoids should be checked in the course of regular physical examinations, and if they become too annoying they can be removed. But surgery for hemorrhoids, it should be noted, is being recommended less and less today as a way to manage this problem.

Blood in Stools

Black, tarry-looking stools may indicate bleeding somewhere in the digestive tract. This can be a symptom of any one of several serious ailments and should be investigated at once by a specialist. Small amounts of blood in stools may not be noticeable, and some outside factors that are harmless may cause the stools to look black. If you are suspicious, kits are available that enable you to conduct a test yourself. Hematest® is one of these that has been around for a long time; kits consist of tissue wipes that you use like toilet paper and simply drop into the toilet to get your reading. These tests are available in drugstores for $5 or $6, or your doctor can give you one.

Instructions that come with the kits must be followed precisely. If you have eaten rare meat recently, you may get a false positive result from the blood in the meat. If you have bleeding hemorrhoids or contaminate the sample with menstrual blood, you will also get a false positive result. On the other hand, if you are taking large amounts of vitamin C, you can get a false negative result. All these instructions and cautions are included with the kits and they are simple to deal with. Several samples should be tested because blood does not disperse evenly in the feces. If you get positive results using one of these tests, further and more extensive tests should be carried out by a doctor at once.

Jaundice and Hepatitis

Yellowing of the skin or of the whites of the eyes may accompany problems with either the liver or the gallbladder and should be given medical attention at once. Some people are plagued with gallstones that don't produce pain but do produce the yellowing effect of jaundice. The yellow pigment won't show up well in dark-complexioned people, of course, so your reliance in this case would be on checking the whites of the eyes. And because you would have a slight amount of pigment in the eye whites under normal circumstances, if you are dark-skinned you should notice and try to remember what your eyes look like when you are well.

The yellowing effect of jaundice is caused by bile backing up in the liver and entering the bloodstream. The kidneys extract the bile and it turns up in the urine. Bile products in the urine can be detected with a variety of dip-and-read urine tests that are available in drugstores. Check with your pharmacist or a medical-supply house. (Also see Chapter 7, "How to Test Your Urinary System.")

Again, instructions that come with the kits must be followed precisely. If you get positive results using one of these tests, further and more extensive tests should be carried out by a doctor at once.

There are two basic causes of jaundice, but whatever the cause, it is a serious situation that shouldn't be ignored. One type is called obstructive jaundice, which occurs when the outflow of bile from the liver to the intestines becomes blocked, either because a gallstone has become lodged in the bile duct or a cancer has formed that is pinching off the duct. The other form of jaundice occurs when the liver cells themselves are not functioning properly, usually as a result of attacks by one of a group of viruses and results in hepatitis.

Hepatitis A is relatively common and is spread by people in a number of ways, but always by ingesting fecally contaminated food or water. It is associated with the *Escherichia coli* bacteria found in stools, which is why when *E. coli* is found in food

or water in large numbers, the assumption is that there is also a danger that hepatitis A is present. Eating uncooked shellfish from contaminated waters is a prime source of hepatitis A. In some parts of the world hepatitis A is virtually endemic, and people who travel to Third World countries should get advice about temporary immunization against this disease. Symptoms of hepatitis A are very similar to flu symptoms, but the addition of jaundice is a telltale clue. You can become quite dramatically ill with hepatitis A, but the cure and recovery rate is nearly 100 percent.

Hepatitis B used to be called blood-borne hepatitis and was often transmitted through blood transfusions. But the most common way of getting hepatitis B these days is through a needle stick. Drug users who share needles are very likely to pass hepatitis B among themselves. Immunization against hepatitis B is widely available, and anyone involved in health care is routinely advised to be immunized.

Hepatitis C presently is not so clearly defined as A and B, and there is no immunization available for it at this time. It is a milder disease during its acute stage but has a high likelihood of becoming chronic. While hepatitis A is more dramatic in its onset, the cure rate is nearly 100 percent, but people do die from B and C.

Involvement of the Nervous System in Poisoning

Visual disturbances followed by muscle weakening and difficulty swallowing are symptoms of botulism, a particularly virulent food poisoning that results from eating improperly canned or prepared food. Symptoms can appear within a few hours or may take days to appear, by which time you may have lost track of what you have eaten. So you may not associate the cause with the effect easily. Food from cans that are bulging, especially noticeable on the ends of the can, or food from containers that explode when you open them, showering some of the contents about, should be avoided. (The explosion is an outward splashing, not the hiss or pop you hear when you open vacuum-sealed nuts or coffee or the pop of a safety seal in the center of the cover on many products.)

Poisonous mushrooms and some kinds of tainted shellfish can also produce symptoms that indicate an effect on the nervous system. Report any such unusual symptoms to a doctor at once; don't wait for the "spell" to pass or go away. Delay can be fatal!

Questions You Should Be Able to Answer

When you have abdominal pain or distress, observe it and track it closely; you may be able to provide vital information to your physician if it comes to that. When did the distress or pain begin? Where is the pain—exactly? Is the pain cramping, dull, sharp, piercing, continuous, intermittent? What other symptoms do you have with the distress? If there is vomiting, diarrhea, or constipation, be able to describe its onset, its appearance, and its frequency.

When you report abdominal distress to the doctor, he or she will probe your abdomen at once. If you have become accustomed to probing your own abdomen under normal circumstances, you will want to do this in times of distress. If you notice swellings or hard spots or enlargements or anything else that seems unusual, report this to the doctor. Sometimes muscle spasms come and go and will not be apparent when the doctor palpates your abdomen; but the information that you felt them can be helpful in making a diagnosis.

Observing and Tracking Bowel Movements

One of the best tests of the gastrointestinal system is simple observation of your bowel movements for size and shape, color, consistency, frequency patterns, and changes that may occur in any of these things. Accurate information describing the past and present status of your bowel movements is a valuable diagnostic tool for your doctor when you complain of abdominal distress or when you are having a general health evaluation, and it is information only you can supply.

Changes are especially important and the only way you can report changes accurately is to make notes in your health record, which spans a period of time. Track your bowel movements and habits for a period of two weeks or so when you feel perfectly well. Track again when you change your diet for one reason or another. Track in times of distress. You will not track for two weeks, of course, in times of obvious distress or when something is plainly wrong—prolonged diarrhea or constipation, signs of bleeding—but any observation that you do have available will be important.

In the event of a change that concerns you, note any recent change in your diet, suspect foods recently eaten, tension or stress you may be experiencing, abdominal pain or distress, whether you have tested your stools for blood and what you have found, and whether changes noticed are recent or long-standing. Record any laxatives, antacids, or other abdominal medicines you are using. Did you recently start taking any prescribed or nonprescribed medications, vitamins, or food supplements?

Generally speaking, people feel better and are more at ease when their bowels are moving regularly and easily. And thanks to commercial exhortations to "regularity," it is something most of us strive for without fully knowing what it is. Daily bowel movements at the same time each day are convenient and commendable but are not all that salutary if they are induced by laxatives on a regular basis. If you take a laxative regularly, in fact, the body adjusts to its presence and it becomes ineffective. A laxative habit, while producing "regularity," can be harmful and of itself is a sign that something is wrong. If you are not happy with the quality and quantity of your stools, try adding fiber to your diet—bran, nuts, raisins, fresh fruits and vegetables, whole-wheat and bran-supplemented breads—and see if it doesn't make a pleasing and dramatic difference.

No one pattern of bowel movements can be called "normal" for everyone. Some people have one bowel movement a day, some have two or more, and some people may normally skip a day, or even two, and then make it up with large quantities on another day. Track your own habits to determine what is normal for you. Frequency of movements may change seasonally as your diet shifts to more fresh foods in the summer or fewer fresh foods in winter. Travel, stress, and inconvenient or dirty toilet facilities can also affect the frequency of your bowel movements. So "regularity" does not tell nearly so much about the state of your digestive tract as the consistency, color, and any changes you may notice in the appearance of your stools.

Observing Bowel Movements

1. Consistency. If stools are dry and hard, they have spent too much time in the colon. If stools are loose and watery, they have been rushed through the colon too fast. If either condition persists, especially when accompanied by abdominal distress or upset, it should be looked into by a physician.

2. Size and shape. The size of stools depends on a person's size and the nature of one's diet. High-fiber diets produce larger, bulkier stools, which seem to be desirable. Narrow, wormlike, or ribbon-shaped stools occur occasionally, but should they persist in this shape, or if they are accompanied by increasing abdominal distress or upset, the condition should be reported to your doctor at once. It could indicate a partial blockage near the end of the colon.

3. Color. Medium brown seems to be the norm for most people. Those on vegetarian diets have lighter-colored stools while meat eaters' are darker. Various foods and medicines may create unusual colors: beets introduce red and may simulate bleeding; iron supplements and Pepto-Bismol make stools black. Black, tarry-looking stools indicate bleeding somewhere in the digestive tract and should be investigated at once. Gray or chalky stools are abnormal and should also be reported to a physician.

4. Change. Change in bowel habits is one of the warning signs of cancer. This is a prime reason for observing and tracking your bowel movements. Temporary or short-lived changes are inevitable, of course, as you eat different foods or experience stomach upsets. Changes may even be long-lasting if they are associated with a permanent change of diet—from low to high fiber, for example. It is persistent change in size, shape, consistency, color, or odor that has no apparent explanation or can't be easily related to a change in diet that you want to watch for.

Tracking Digestive Upsets of Indeterminate Cause

Many people endure chronic indigestion, constipation, or diarrhea that persists, with no apparent reason, even after a thorough medical evaluation has been conducted. Diagnoses are sometimes of "stress," "irritable colon," or some other vagueness that

means "there doesn't seem to be anything wrong organically so it must be something in your diet or your job or nervousness or something like that." Sometimes when a doctor explains this and exhorts the patient to calm down, symptoms disappear.

In situations of unexplained and unexplainable distress, it may help to keep a diary of distressful episodes and see if a pattern emerges. Record the date and time, foods eaten, drugs being used (including tobacco and alcohol), and whether you have been tense or nervous (record the circumstances) and make any comments that seem relevant.

Some people quickly discover this way that bouts of diarrhea quickly follow drinking milk or eating ice cream. Indigestion, constipation, or diarrhea may follow or precede going on trips, family quarrels, or stress on the job. But if nothing else, you will amass a useful record for the doctor to analyze on your next visit.

Pinworms

Pinworms are tiny white worms that inhabit the lower end of the large intestine. Either adults or children may become infected with the worms, but children are generally the first in a family to get them. If you suspect your child has pinworms, you should look carefully in the anal region either very late at night after the child has been asleep for several hours or very early in the morning before the child awakens. You may be able to actually see the tiny worms before they crawl back into the bowel through the anal sphincter after laying their eggs.

More often than not, however, the pin-worms are not caught at the moment they have come out to lay eggs. The diagnosis of pinworm disease, therefore, rests on finding pinworm eggs. These are tiny little eggs that are microscopic in size. A pinworm egg test is relatively simple, but you must have a microscope to carry it out. Most home microscopes or those used in high school laboratories will do.

Testing for Pinworms

1. Take a piece of cellophane tape and blot it around the skin surrounding the child's anus first thing in the morning before the child gets out of bed.

2. Place the piece of tape on a microscope slide, sticky side down.

3. Examine the slide using the high-magnification lens on your microscope. The tape picks up a large number of dirt particles, loose skin cells, small hairs, and almost anything else that is loose in the area, including pinworm eggs. Pinworm

eggs, however, are a very characteristic shape and once you see one there will be no doubt in your mind that you have found it. A pinworm egg is about the same oval shape as a hen's egg; it is clear and when viewed under the microscope a tiny worm can be seen folded up inside.

For pinworms to grow, the egg must somehow be transmitted to the mouth of another person. This may seem difficult at first, but because eggs are only microscopic in size and very light, they can flow through the air attached to dust particles and can easily settle on food, dishes, and even someone's toothbrush.

If a child is continually scratching his or her bottom, pinworms can be one reason. If any member of the family contracts a pinworm infestation, the bed linen and pajamas for everyone should be washed simultaneously, there should be a general house cleaning, and everyone in the household should be simultaneously treated by a physician, who will likely prescribe a single dose of medicine that will take care of the problem in most cases.

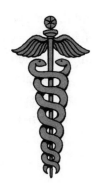

4

How to Test Your Vision

In the days before television, the way the eyes work was best described in terms of the famous Brownie box camera, and as far as it goes, the analogy is still a good one. Both eye and camera are enclosed receptacles with a small hole in front to admit light rays. Both have a diaphragm to regulate the amount of light entering the optical system and both have a lens that focuses the light on a light-sensitive film. The energy in the light causes chemical changes in the film of the camera, and chemical changes also occur when light strikes what are called rods and cones on the light-sensitive "film" or retina at the back of the eye. This is, very simply speaking, how light images are received in the eye.

But when it comes to seeing, it helps to think of the eye more in terms of a television camera, where the images received are translated into electrical impulses that are transmitted via cable to a screen where a picture is produced instantaneously. In the eye, chemical changes in the rods and cones,

caused by the energy in light rays, are translated into electrical impulses that are transmitted along a cable—the optic nerve—to the brain that interprets the impulses and allows you to see a picture, instantaneously, of what you are looking at.

The difference between the eyes and a television camera is that the eye-brain combination is a much more sophisticated system. Eyes have automatic synchronization, focusing, diaphragm control, and interpretation features that are far beyond the capabilities of the best TV equipment. And the eyes have built-in maintenance systems to boot.

The entrance to the eye is covered by a clear, slightly dome-shaped structure called the cornea. The cornea is so clear that it can't be seen easily when you look directly into your eyes, so if you would like to get a good look at your cornea, stand close to a mirror and shine a small flashlight onto the colored part of your eye from the side. The clear cornea can easily be seen looking like a spherical cap or watch crystal over the colored part of the eye and the black hole, or pupil, in the center.

The cornea is the first part of the focusing system that light strikes as it enters the eye. Being in the very front of the eyes, the corneas are very vulnerable to injuries that can cause severe loss of vision or blindness—a good reason to see that your eyes are well protected when working in potentially dangerous situations.

The amount of light entering the eye is controlled by the iris—the colored part—which is equivalent to the diaphragm in a camera. When there is more light than the eye likes, the iris makes the pupil, or eye opening, smaller. In dim light, the iris draws back, enlarging the pupil to admit as much light as possible. This is an automatic response, or reflex action, and it is one of several reflexes that a doctor looks at when performing a general examination of a patient.

Testing Pupillary Reflex

1. Looking into a mirror, shine the light from a small flashlight into the eye diagonally, from the outside corner. Do not

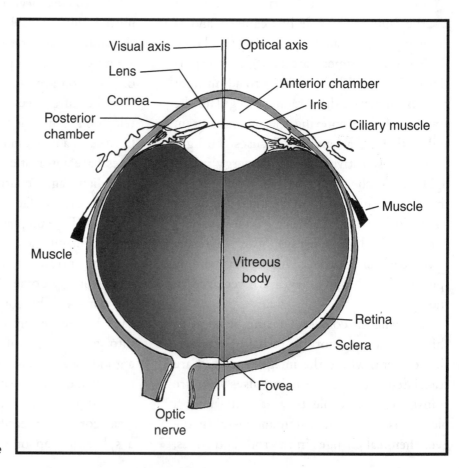

Inside the Eye

shine the light directly into your eye, and a momentary flash of light will do.

2. As the light strikes your eye you will see the iris instantly contract to make the pupil smaller. When you take the light away, the pupil becomes instantly larger. This pupillary reflex should be strong and rapid.

Certain diseases and injuries can affect the proper functioning of the irises so that they do not respond to changes in light the way they should. In these cases, the pupils may not change in size when light shines in the eyes, or the pupils may appear to be unequal in size. Drugs can also affect the irises' response to light. Heavy doses of opium-derived drugs such as codeine and heroin can cause pinpoint-sized pupils, and this is one sign that doctors or law-enforcement officers look for when they suspect they are dealing with someone who has recently used these drugs. Other drugs affect the iris in such a way that the pupil openings become quite large. An old drug, belladonna, is one of these and, in fact, got its name from just this phenomenon. *Bella donna* means "beautiful woman," and at a time when large pupils and a delicate skin pallor were considered alluring, women would use the drug to create these conditions. But if they did use belladonna cosmetically, the ladies must have suffered for their beauty, because the drug causes some uncomfortable side effects, including blurred vision and an oppressively dry mouth.

As light rays pass the iris they encounter the lens of the eye, where they are focused sharply toward the retina at the back of the eye. The eye must adjust to focus images on the retina, whether the object being looked at is nearby or far away. This happens in a camera when the photographer slightly changes the distance between the lens and the film plane. The photographer's other choice is to change the strength of the lens, and this is accomplished by adding different lenses for objects very near or very far away from the camera.

The eye accommodates itself to seeing objects at different distances by increasing and decreasing the power of its lens. Muscles around the lens contract to make the lens thicker and its focal length shorter. In a normal eye light from objects eighteen feet or more away will focus on the retina while the muscles around the lens are at rest. Then, when you look at objects closer than eighteen feet, the muscles contract to make the lens thicker, which shortens the focus, and an image is formed again exactly on the retina. This is why it is more tiring to do close work than it is to search the horizon for ships at sea. The muscles around the lens must work harder when you do close work.

When the optical system of the eye cannot focus light precisely on the retina for one reason or another, the image formed is slightly blurred and you need corrective eyeglasses or contact lenses. How well you see is usually spoken of in terms of visual acuity. Visual acuity is the ability to see one object as distinct from another and recognize it. Thus, if you can read the letters on a sign down the street and your friend can't, you have the better visual acuity.

Visual Acuity

No two people see just alike and there is a fairly wide range of what is considered normal vision. But certain arbitrary standards have been set that are a good guide to how well one person can see in relation to another. The familiar chart with letters that get progressively smaller line by line is the most common test used in general screening for visual acuity at distances of more than eighteen feet. The chart used most often is called the Snellen scale. Eye-test charts can be obtained inexpensively from most medical-supply stores or by contacting Prevent Blindness America, 500 East Remington Road, Schaumburg, IL 60173; 800-331-2020. There are special E charts and picture charts for preschoolers and those who cannot read.

Distance Vision

Eye-test charts are designed to be used at a distance of twenty feet. This gives the first part of the visual acuity rating: 20/20, 20/30, 20/40, and so on. The second or third smallest line of letters from the bottom will be labeled 20/20. If you can read this line of letters easily and accurately, it means that you see as clearly at twenty feet as most people do whose vision is considered normal. If you can read only as far down the chart as the line labeled 20/30, this means that at twenty feet you are only able to see what most people with normal vision can see at thirty feet. If you can read only the line labeled 20/200 when you

are standing twenty feet away from the chart, it means your vision is rather severely limited because most people with normal vision can see these letters from 200 feet away.

Going in the opposite direction, if you can read the tiny 20/15 line, your distance vision is a bit sharper than it is for most people.

Testing Visual Acuity

1. Place the eye chart in good light and position yourself twenty feet away from it. (Charts are available to use at ten feet with a good mirror to produce a reflected image that is twenty feet away.) Be sure there are no shadows and no glare on the chart.

2. Cover one eye gently with a card or your cupped hand. Don't press on the eye you are covering.

3. Read the smallest line of letters you can see clearly. Have someone close to the chart check to see that you are not stumbling over letters or reading them incorrectly. Record the label of the smallest line you can read.

4. Switch eyes and do the same thing. This time read the line backward to be sure you are not reading from memory.

5. Finally, test with both eyes open.

If you are not experiencing any discomfort when you use your eyes, a test score as low as 20/40 is generally considered adequately good vision for most purposes, although some occupations require better than 20/40 vision or vision that can be brought to 20/20 with corrective lenses. Police and fire departments and the military services are among those that usually require better visual acuity. If you score worse than 20/40, you should visit an eye doctor for a formal evaluation. If your eyes test in the normal range but one eye tests considerably better than the other, say 20/20 for one and 20/40 for the other, you should also get a professional evaluation.

A Rough Test for Distance Vision

A rough but effective way to check the quality of distance vision is simply to compare your ability to read road signs or billboard advertising with someone who is known to have good vision. It can be made a game with children. Predetermine the distance at which a clearly lettered sign is just visible to the person with good vision. Have the person being tested try to read the words with one eye at a time. If there is noticeable difficulty—that is, if the person being tested has to move a good bit closer to the sign than seems necessary—more formal testing should be conducted.

People are often confused about the labels attached to various eye-care professionals. These are the differences:

- Ophthalmologist. An ophthalmologist has an M.D. with a specialty in diseases of the eye. The ophthalmologist can treat any condition of the eye, from simple mechanical difficulties that require eyeglasses or contact lenses to diseases requiring medication or surgery.

- Optometrist. An optometrist holds a degree of Doctor of Optometry, O.D., from a school of optometry. He or she primarily treats mechanical problems of the eye and prescribes eyeglasses or contact lenses. An optometrist is well trained, however, in the anatomy and physiology of the eye and is able to recognize diseases. He or she will refer you to an ophthalmologist for any condition that he or she discovers which requires medical treatment. Many ophthalmologists today include optometrists in their practice for their skill in using eye-testing optical equipment.

- Optician. An optician is a craftsman who sells and fits eyeglasses and contact lenses from a prescription provided by an ophthalmologist or optometrist.

- Oculist. This is an older term that is no longer used because it was too loosely applied to any practitioner who had anything to do with the eyes.

Blurred distance vision is more often the result of an error in the eye's optical system than a result of a defect in the nerves, blood vessels, or other tissues that serve the eye. The eyeball itself may be a bit too long in relation to the strength of the lens system so that light from distant objects focuses short of the retina. This is what happens in myopia, or nearsightedness. In nearsightedness, as the name implies, distance vision is not so good as it should be and this can be spotted easily with eye-chart testing.

Another error in the optical system, which often goes unnoticed in young people, is hyperopia, or farsightedness. In hyperopia, light tries to focus behind the retina. But this signals the muscles around the lens to shorten the focus, which they do by squeezing the lens to make it a bit thicker. This corrects the error and allows the hyperope to see 20/20 or better, but it keeps the muscles working overtime and can result in fatigue and headaches. With aging, however, a hyperope may begin to experience blurred distance vision because, as one gets older, the accommodation mechanism becomes progressively more inefficient. This blurring will show up—in older people, not in young people—with eye-chart testing.

Near Vision

In addition to testing your vision at twenty feet, you should measure your *near point of accommodation*. This is the closest point in front of your eyes where you can see an object clearly without blurring or distortion. If you do a good bit of close work—reading, writing, sewing, sorting, assembling, repairing—and if you are approaching forty, it is important for you to understand this near point and to know where it is for you.

Determining Your Near Point of Accommodation

1. To find your near point, take an ordinary yardstick and rest its end gently against your cheekbone. Hold the yardstick so that it sticks out directly in front of you.

2. Hold some reading material with fairly small print in the other hand. A newspaper, magazine, or this book will do. Hold the reading material at a distance along the yardstick where you can read the words easily.

3. Move the page toward you, watching the letters as they become more difficult to read. At some point the words will blur and become difficult to read. Move the page back out until you can read the words comfortably again. Note where this point is on the yardstick. This distance from your eye to the page is your near point of accommodation.

If you are under forty, your near point should be about twelve to fourteen inches or closer. In young people the near point can be as close as three or four inches. If you are past forty and are already wearing a corrective prescription for reading—either reading glasses or bifocals—your near point should also be within a twelve- to fourteen-inch range or shorter when you are wearing your glasses. When the near point moves out beyond fourteen inches, as it does inexorably with aging, it becomes inconvenient, uncomfortable, and sometimes dangerous to work without corrective lenses. It is foolhardy to work around fast-moving machinery, for instance, if you are not sure you can see it clearly at a comfortable working distance. And a day at the office can be sheer misery if you must struggle constantly to find a distance at which you can see your work.

The condition is called presbyopia and it happens to everyone. It is a result of the progressing inefficiency of the accommodation mechanism of the eye mentioned earlier. Reading glasses or a reading correction added to a prescription you already wear (bifocals) easily solves the problem. If your work requires constant shifting of your eyes from near to intermediate to distant objects, such as a teacher might have to do in shifting from blackboard to students to a book, trifocal lenses that help focus light from three distances are often a practical solution. Various combinations of contact and reading glasses also work well. Discuss the options with your eye doctor.

In young people the near point is generally not much of a concern, although what happens when a young person does near work is important. We noted that young, farsighted (hyperopic) people can usually see quite well at a distance, but their eye muscles are under constant tension to put images on the retina. The closer the object, the harder the muscles must work. So reading and other near work can put considerably more strain on farsighted eyes than on normal eyes. This will not be noticed as blurred vision; but fatigue, headache, dizziness, and nausea after periods of close work may tip you off that something is amiss. Children with this condition are usually unaware that anything is wrong, but they become understandably reluctant to read or do other near work. Whenever there is

undue reluctance to read or do schoolwork, vision should be checked by an eye doctor as a possible cause.

Most people do not have their visual acuity and other functions of seeing checked as often as they should. Children should have their first professional eye examination no later than age three and preferably younger. Certain defects can be corrected only if they are discovered and treated when a child is very young. Eyes should be tested again when a child starts school and then at two-year intervals throughout life. Where adults are concerned, such things as retinal detachments and glaucoma are treated today with extremely high success rates when they are discovered early. When they go undiscovered and untreated, they quickly cause irreversible eye damage.

Visual screening for near and distance vision should be a part of the health program in every school. If there is no program in your child's school, you may want to contact Prevent Blindness America, referred to earlier, for information and help in getting one started. With very little training, volunteer nonprofessionals can conduct highly effective visual-screening programs.

Astigmatism

Astigmatism is another common problem that occurs in the eye's optical system. What happens in astigmatism is that light rays from objects in different planes of vision focus at different points within the eye. That is, when you look at the letter E on the eye chart or on a road sign, for example, you may see the vertical bar of the E more clearly than the crossbars; or one line of an X may look clearer and darker than the other. This is generally attributed to an error in the shape of the cornea or in the shape of the eyeball itself. Both blurring and distortion can occur with astigmatism and may result in obvious discomfort—headaches, tension, tightness—as the eyes try to cope with focusing different images in different planes.

Testing for Astigmatism

1. Many cases of astigmatism can be discerned with a simple eye chart you can make yourself. On white paper draw eight pairs of lines that are forty-five degrees apart and pointing at a common center, as shown in the illustration. This results in a sort of circular clock face.

Make the lines about eight inches long and about ¼ inch wide. Use a black felt-tip pen or marking crayon and be sure that all the lines are equally wide and equally black.

2. Place the chart in good light about twenty feet away. If you can't see the chart at twenty feet, move closer until you can see the lines. Cover one eye and see if any set of lines looks darker, clearer, or sharper than the set of lines at right angles to it. Repeat with the other eye. If there seems to be a distinct difference in the darkness and clarity of one set of lines over that at right angles to it, then some degree of astigmatism probably exists and a professional evaluation is in order. Most astigmatism can be corrected easily with eyeglasses.

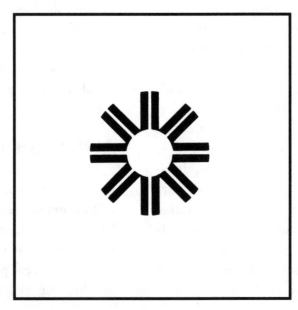

A Test for Astigmatism

Coordination of Eye Movements

While the optical system of the eye is a genuine wonder by itself, even more wonderful is the rapid communication between the eyes and the brain that enables us to see the world as we do and perform a variety of functions, which, if you stop to think about them, should really be impossible. You can look at an object and know if it is near or far away and you can estimate its size at any distance. You can judge textures, from big bumps on the earth called mountains to the little bumps that make the difference between sheer and nubby curtain material.

This happens, in part, because of the brain's ability to change two-dimensional images received by the eyes into three-dimensional visual perception. We say, then, that we have depth perception and the world has form and texture for us because of it. People with only one eye can have an adequate sense of depth and they can judge distances, but it works much better with two eyes—binocular vision, this is called.

Because the eyes are separated, each sees a slightly different image, and the brain fuses these into a single, three-dimensional picture. Another feature of binocular vision is the ability of the eyes to move in their sockets in synchronized and coordinated movements in response to either conscious or unconscious commands from the brain. Both these phenomena are easy to observe.

Testing Eye Coordination

1. Have the person being tested sit holding his or her head steady, looking straight forward.

2. Ask your subject to follow the motion of your hand with his or her eyes, without moving his or her head, as you move your hand up and down, from side to side, diagonally, and, finally, in a circle. The range of motion of the eyes, which is controlled by six paired and opposing muscles in each eye, is quite remarkable.

3. Then, ask your subject to watch your finger as you move it from a distance to the tip of his or her nose. The eyes turn in and down, a movement that is much more obvious in younger people, who can fixate on an object as close as two or three inches from the eyes.

4. Now, hold your finger steady a foot or more away and ask your subject to look at it while moving the head up and down, sideways, and in a circle. Now the eyes remain in one position while the eye sockets and the rest of the head revolve around them. The same muscles are at work.

Observe these eye movements carefully. The eyes should work together smoothly. Especially notice what happens when you move your finger from far to near and back out again. One eye may turn slightly more than the other, or at least the turning may be more noticeable in one eye than in the other. But if there are large differences in the movements—one eye turns considerably more than the other, one refuses to turn or follows reluctantly—there may be a muscle imbalance or coordination problem that should be noted and discussed in the course of a professional eye examination.

To prove that your eyes see different images, hold up your finger and, with one eye closed, align the finger with a distant object. Now switch eyes. The relationship between finger and object shifts noticeably. Open and close your eyes alternately and there is a good bit of jumping around of images.

Generally, one eye is a fixing or dominant eye, while the other obediently turns to fix on the same object the dominant eye is looking at. If this doesn't happen, you may get double vision. Double vision can result from a variety of causes that include too much alcohol, fatigue, muscle imbalance, defects in the eyes' optical system, and perception problems that originate in the brain. Any condition that indicates that the eyes are not working together to see a single image should be reported to the doctor at once.

Finding Your Dominant Eye

Most people have a dominant right eye just as most people have a dominant right hand. And what's more, chances are good that your dominant eye will be on the same side as your dominant hand.

1. Cut a circle in the center of a piece of paper or in an index card. About a one-inch circle will do, and it doesn't have to be perfectly round.

2. Hold the circle about a foot away from your eyes, and with both eyes open, sight through the circle at some distant object.

3. Hold your index finger so that it lines up with the center of the hole and the object you are sighting on—like sighting a rifle at a target.

4. Close your left eye. If the circle, your finger, and the object are still lined up, you are sighting or fixing with your right eye. If the opposite is true, if everything is lined up with the left eye open and the right eye shut, you are sighting with your left eye.

Strabismus

When the two eyes fail to turn and work together, the condition is known as strabismus. This and other conditions, such as when one eye has much better visual acuity than the other, often cause the brain to suppress vision in one of the eyes. Rather than deal with disparate and confusing images, the brain may prefer to "turn off" one of the pictures. Most people can do this voluntarily when sighting a rifle or when looking through a magnifying glass with one eye only, although both eyes are kept open.

If the brain persistently suppresses the vision in one eye during normal seeing, the suppressed eye will eventually lose its ability to see. This happens more often than it should with young children. Many parents, noticing that a child's eyes are not working together, simply wait for the child to "outgrow" it. This attitude arises from the fact that infants' eyes tend to dissociate, or not work together, up to about six months, and then they do outgrow it. But after six months, the eyes should be developed enough to work together, and if they don't the condition should be investigated at once. Vision in a suppressed eye can be lost fairly rapidly, so the sooner it is caught the better. Treatment for this condition is faster and more successful if begun before age three and success rates decline markedly after that. Many ophthalmologists suggest a professional eye examination in infancy and again before age three. And certainly any noticeable crossing or divergence in children's eyes should be investigated at once.

Visual Field

At the beginning of this chapter we pointed out that light impulses are picked up and started on their way to the brain by specialized cells called rods and cones that are located on the retina—the light-sensitive "film" at the back of the eye. The retina is about the size of a postage stamp, as thin as onionskin, and loaded with rods and cones, perhaps 150 million or more of them. Rods can only perceive images as black and white, while cones can discern color.

The most sensitive point on the retina is a small spot near the center called the fovea, which is barely one-fiftieth of an inch in diameter and packed with cones. It is here that the sharpest vision and most color vision occurs. The eyes stay in constant motion, even when you're not aware of it, in an effort

to keep the image of whatever you are looking at focused on this tiny spot.

With one eye closed, stare at the second *n* in the word concentrate. You will see the *e* and the *t* on either side of the *n* rather well, but you will notice that letters beyond that quickly begin to get gray and fade. Your area of sharpest vision and best color discrimination is quite small. But beyond that the total field of vision is surprisingly large, even though you see only in black and white over most of it. You can see almost straight to the side—out of the "corner" of your eye—while looking straight ahead, and you could do as well up and down and to the other side if it weren't for eyebrows, cheekbones, and your nose getting in the way. Because there are diseases of both the eyes themselves and the brain that tend to reduce the extent of this visual field, it is important that you are familiar with what it is and how far it extends for you. You can do this very simply.

Testing Your Visual Field

1. Stand a little more than arm's length away from a wall with your right shoulder pointing toward some convenient marker on the wall, such as the edge of a picture.

2. Choose a small object directly in front of you and some distance away, and stare at it intently. Cover your left eye with your left hand.

3. Now, hold your right hand out from your right side on a level with your eyes and pointing at your mark on the wall.

4. Move your arm just back from the mark and point your fingers forward loosely. Wiggle your fingers and slowly move your arm forward. Continue staring intently at the object in front of you. Resist the temptation to peek at your fingers.

5. After you move your arm just slightly forward, your wiggling fingers will suddenly come into view even as you are staring straight to the front. This will not be a sharp image, but the motion will be clearly perceived. This is the edge of your visual field on your right side using the right eye.

6. Stop as soon as you hit this point and look to see where your arm is. It should be about 80° or 85° from a line straight in front of you—about 15° from the mark on the wall. Touch the wall. You will be less than six inches from your marker. This means you can perceive objects almost directly to the side but not quite.

7. Perform the same test with your wiggling fingers from several angles—above your head, from below, diagonally, and from the nose side. (You will have to change hands when working from the

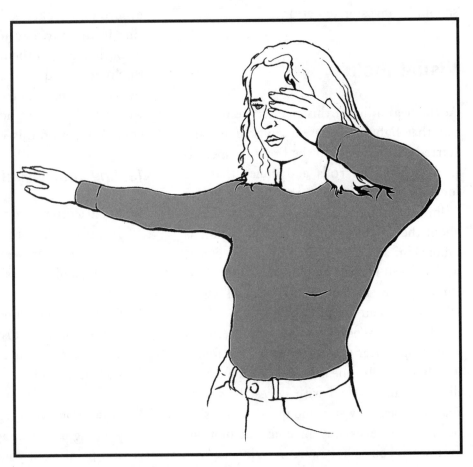

Position for Testing Visual Field

nasal side.) The field from above will only be about 50° and just a little better from the bottom. This is because your eyebrows and cheekbones are in the way. You will manage still less from the side where the nose gets in the way. Test both eyes in the same manner.

The importance of your field of vision is obvious in avoiding danger from the side when driving an automobile, in performing well in sports, and in many occupations that require you to be aware of what's going on at the edges of your visual field. But most important, a contracting visual field can be a sign of major trouble and must be investigated by an eye doctor as soon as it is suspected. Check the edges of your visual field at least once a year. If your field seems to be shrinking, even by a small amount, call this to the attention of an eye specialist to determine what is going on.

Your Blind Spot

Light impulses are carried from the retina of the eye to the brain in a bundle of nerves called the optic nerve. The point at which the optic nerve enters the eyeball is called the optic disc. The disc is like the end of an electric cable with a large number of wires (nerves) being sent out from it to points on the retina where they make contact with the photoreceptor cells (rods and cones). The optic disc itself contains no rods or cones and is, therefore, a blind spot. Everyone has two blind spots, one in each eye. A normal blind spot never gives any trouble in seeing: We're never even aware of it, in fact, but there is an amusing trick that proves it is there.

Blind-Spot Demonstration

1. Make a ½-inch-diameter black spot on a piece of stiff paper—a 3 × 5 index card works fine. About three inches to the left of the spot make a star, or just an *x* will do.

2. Close your left eye and hold the paper at arm's length with the star directly in front of your right eye. Stare fixedly at the star (or *x*) and bring the paper slowly toward your face. At some point the black spot will disappear. The reason it disappears is that the image of the spot has fallen on the blind spot of your right eye.

3. Move the paper a bit closer and the spot reappears. To find the blind spot of your left eye, stare at the spot with the right eye closed and make the star disappear in the same way.

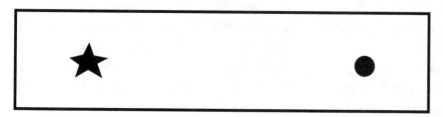

Blind-Spot Demonstration

Retinal Detachment and Glaucoma

Of the conditions that can cause a progressive loss of vision, retinal detachment and glaucoma are most worthy of mention here simply because they can be treated so successfully when discovered in time. Retinal detachments can result from disease, injury, or from less obvious and sometimes mysterious causes. The retina separates from the back of the eye with resulting blindness where the detachment occurs. Modern treatment of this disease has been well covered in the press because of its space-age technology involving the use of cryosurgery (freezing) and laser beams. And success rates are as spectacular as the techniques—as high as 90 percent when the condition is discovered and treatment begun in time. Seeing showers of spots or shadows, seeing cuts or black bars, or a sudden and noticeable decrease in the field of vision should be investigated at once.

Some spots people see, usually after age fifty, are normal. These are specks that float in the vitreous, the fluid that fills the eyeball to help maintain its shape. These "floaters" cast shadows on the retina and are always moving around. The first time you notice them they are both annoying and alarming. These are usually benign, but because they can sometimes occur with other more serious problems, you should have them checked promptly by an ophthalmologist when they first appear.

Glaucoma is an insidious eye disease that has been called "the thief of sight." Of two million Americans who have the disease, it is estimated that half are unaware of it, which is a terrible statistic considering that glaucoma can almost always be kept in check easily with eyedrops, but if left alone it can cause irreversible blindness.

About four-fifths of the eyeball is filled with a clear jellylike material, the vitreous humor, that exerts just the right amount of pressure to enable the eye to keep its shape. In the very front part of the eye this material is thin and watery and is referred to as the aqueous humor. There is constant circulation of the aqueous humor with new material secreted as some of it is drained off. If the secretion rate exceeds the drainage rate, pressure within the eye increases. This is what happens in glaucoma. If the condition is allowed to continue without treatment, the pressure will destroy the delicate retina with resulting blindness.

Deterioration of vision associated with glaucoma is likely to begin around the edge of the visual field, usually starting from the nasal side of the eye. But defects in the field do not necessarily progress in a constant fashion, and large cuts in the visual field can occur before the defect is noticed if formal testing is not conducted on a regular basis. Then, even though the disease is brought under control, the vision that has been lost is gone permanently.

The best test for glaucoma is a direct measurement of the pressure inside the eyeball, which is done with an instrument called a tonometer. Tonometer testing should be performed only by a doctor or other specially trained person; it is not recommended for home testing. Because glaucoma is much more common in people over the age of forty-five, people approaching the middle years should be tested regularly with a tonometer, just as they should be tested regularly with an electrocardiograph to check on the heart. This is why having your eyes checked by an eye specialist at least every two years, or more often, is recommended even if you feel your visual acuity has not changed.

The Lions Club International, which has been interested in sight preservation for many years, has begun a program of free tonometer testing in some communities. You might want to contact the Lions Club in your area to find out if it has a program.

Cataract

Cataract is a disease that affects the eyes of many older people. Some conditions cause cataracts in young people—such as congenital cataracts in infants that may result from a mother having had German measles during pregnancy—but the majority of cataracts occur in people over sixty. A cataract is a clouding of the lens of the eye that generally develops over a period of years, although some are known to develop in a matter of months. It begins as a very mild turbidity in the lens, perhaps in just a spot or two, and then as time goes on the lens admits less and less light into the eye. This will result in hazy vision that is likely to show up in eye-chart testing, or it will simply become apparent that sight is not so sharp as it used to be. Night driving may become increasingly difficult because light from approaching cars is diffused by the cloudiness in the lens, producing a dazzling effect.

The exact mechanism that results in cataract is unknown and the treatment consists of surgically removing the cloudy lens. It is an operation that is performed routinely with little risk and only a brief hospital stay. Then, with the help of a plastic lens implant, glasses, or contact lenses, vision is dramatically restored.

Conjunctivitis

Almost everyone, at some point, has had an experience where the whites of the eyes and the linings of the eyelids become red and inflamed-looking. Because of the redness, you sometimes hear the condition referred to as pinkeye. A discharge may crust and stick the eyelids together when you wake up in the morning. Often there is itching and the feeling that there is something in the eye. These are classic symptoms of conjunctivitis.

The conjunctiva is a mucous membrane that lines the eyelids and the white part of the eye. The conjunctiva can become infected or inflamed from a viral or bacterial invasion (swimming is a common culprit here), from allergies, and from exposure to irritating chemicals. Your primary-care physician can take care of this condition easily with antibiotics, or allergy medication if an allergy is the cause, and you should not put off having it taken care of.

Redness of the eyelid, burning, tearing, and the feeling of something in the eye may also presage the coming of a sty—a small, hard boil that forms at the base of an eyelash. This is usually treated with antibiotic medication and, at the recommendation and direction of a doctor, hot compresses may help.

Corneal Injuries

The cornea—the clear, dome-shaped structure over the pupil and iris at the front of the eye—is the first part of the eye's optical system that light encounters, and it is the first part of the eye that is subject to injury from flying debris. That's why every power tool you buy warns about wearing safety goggles (ordinary eyeglasses don't provide protection), and many tools now come with safety glasses included as part of the package. Use them! Corneal injuries tend to form scar tissue that inhibits vision. If you do get something lodged in the cornea, or in the white part of the eye, you must see an ophthalmologist at once.

Summary

Everyone should become familiar with their eyes—how they see and what normal eyes look like. Any unusual condition should be called to the attention of a doctor. Here, in summary, are the most common:

- Unusual sensitivity to light
- Persistent pain, burning, or itching
- Headaches associated with using the eyes
- Redness of the eyeball; marks or bumps
- Anything unusual about the eyelids, inside or outside
- Excessive tearing or unusual discharges; eyelids that stick together
- Change in pupil size; unequal pupil sizes: very large or very small pupils
- Seeing halos when you look at lights
- Poor night vision
- Seeing black bands, shadows, spots, or anything else that shouldn't be there
- Shrinking visual field (developing tunnel vision)
- Double vision

The visual acuity test, using the letter chart, is the most useful tool for a quick general-vision evaluation. If your vision is poorer than the 20/20 to 20/40 range, you should consult an eye doctor. The other tests we have described are extremely useful in keeping track of your eyes over the years and between the times that you see your doctor. But if you develop any of the untoward symptoms described previously, consult an eye doctor. In the case of glaucoma, retinal detachments, and certain other conditions delay in consulting a doctor can result in irretrievable vision loss that could have been prevented.

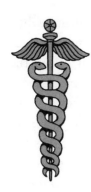

5

Tests of Your Ears, Nose, Throat, and Mouth

The nose, mouth, and throat are essentially a single chamber divided by partitions at various places and at various angles. The ear is connected to this chamber via a little tube called the Eustachian tube, which runs from the middle ear to the back of the throat. Because of these interconnecting passageways, an infection in one part of the chamber is easily spread to adjacent areas. That's why the common cold can affect you with a sore throat, a stuffy nose, and, if you blow too hard, an ear infection all at the same time.

You can perform a variety of tests to check the ears, nose, mouth, and throat. Most of them require a minimum of professional equipment, and some consist simply of knowing what to look for. You may find it worthwhile, however, to purchase an otoscope for your medical-supplies kit, particularly if you or someone in your family has a history of ear infections.

An otoscope is a small, hand-held instrument that enables an examiner to peer into the external ear canal or nasal cavity. It is the first instrument a doctor uses in a general physical examination to peer into the various openings in your head. This can be a valuable aid in identifying abnormal conditions that require medical attention. The device consists of a little funnel that is placed in the ear or nose, a light arranged in such a way that it shines down the center of the funnel, and a lens that magnifies whatever there is to be seen at the far end of the funnel. A serviceable instrument suitable for home use can be purchased from medical-supply houses for about $30, depending on the brand and model. Some perfectly serviceable otoscopes can sometimes be found in drugstores and mail-order catalogs for even less.

Should you go shopping for an otoscope, you may be shown kits consisting of a handle containing batteries and a switch, interchangeable otoscope and ophthalmoscope heads, different size funnels for different size ear canals as well as for the broader nasal openings, and a handsome carrying case. The ophthalmoscope head is for looking into the eyes and from the point of view of the home observer is not particularly useful. Because it is possible to purchase the component parts individually, you would be better advised to save your money on the ophthalmoscope head and the carrying case and buy only the handle, the otoscope head (some convert to a throat illuminator), and the assorted funnels.

The Ears

Before actually examining the ear, it is helpful to understand how the ear is constructed and what you are likely to find when you go looking.

The ear is anatomically divided into three sections: the outer, or external, ear, the middle ear, and the inner ear. The outer ear consists of a shell-like, cartilaginous flap that acts as a funnel, catching sounds and channeling them into the external auditory canal. This quarter-inch-wide canal runs a little more than an inch inside the head and is sealed off at its inner end by a cone-shaped membrane known as the eardrum. You should be able to see the eardrum using an otoscope by following the instructions presented further on in this chapter. This membrane, of course, effectively obstructs any view of the middle and inner ear.

The middle ear consists of a small cavity containing a chain of three minuscule bones, called the hammer, the anvil, and the stirrup because of their fanciful resemblance to these objects. One end of this chain—the ham-

mer—makes contact with the eardrum, while the other end—the stirrup—communicates with the inner ear via an organ called the cochlea. The spiral-shaped cochlea is about a quarter inch across at its base and contains the auditory nerve endings that transmit sound to the brain. The brain decodes the myriad sounds that are fed to it through the auditory nerve and converts them into meaningful messages. The cochlea together with the three semicircular canals, which help with balance, constitute the inner ear.

Because the middle ear is sealed in by the eardrum, air-pressure differences would build up within this cavity if it did not have some other connection to the outside world. This connection is provided by a slender tube called the Eustachian tube, which extends from the middle ear into the throat. Its function is to equalize pressure on both sides of the eardrum. If the pressure on the outside of the eardrum changes for any reason—a loud noise, a change in atmospheric pressure, a ride in an elevator or an airplane—the pressure within the middle ear must adjust to that on the outside. If pressure equalization does not occur, we say that our ears are plugged up, and we cannot hear properly until they become unplugged. Most of us have experienced this feeling when riding in an airplane or driving in the mountains. To "unplug" our ears, we swallow. This action automatically opens the Eustachian tube, thus providing the middle ear with access to the outside world and a means of regulating air pressure on both sides of the eardrum.

A similar situation occurs when the middle ear becomes infected. The infection

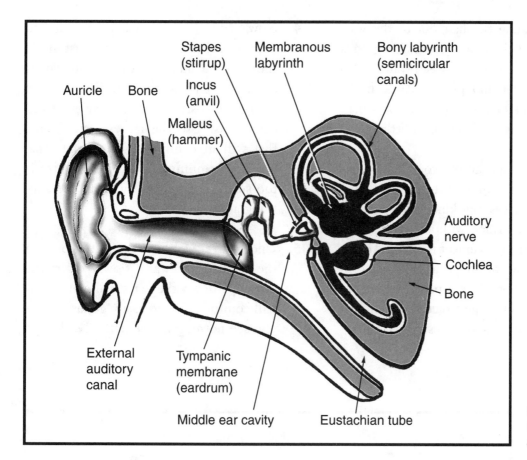

Organs of the Outer, Middle, and Inner Ear

itself is usually not particularly painful. But when it clogs the slender Eustachian tube leading down to the throat, pressure builds up in the middle ear, producing a feeling of acute discomfort. The doctor will treat the infection, of course, and may prescribe a decongestant.

Using an Otoscope

The only part of the ear available for direct inspection is the outer ear. This includes the external auditory canal and the eardrum itself. As noted earlier in this chapter, an otoscope is a valuable aid in examining the outer ear. If you have invested in an otoscope, here is how you use it. You cannot, of course, examine your own ears with an otoscope. You will have to look at someone else's ears and someone else will have to look at yours. But before you use your otoscope, ask your doctor to demonstrate the technique on your next visit.

1. To use the otoscope, the subject should either be seated or lying down with the head resting comfortably against a pillow, a high-backed chair, or a wall. The subject's head should be turned somewhat to bring the ear forward for easy examination.

2. First, brushing the hair out of the way, take hold of the rear of the cartilaginous shell of the outer ear between your thumb and forefinger and pull it firmly backward. This straightens out the ear canal, which is normally bent just a little.

3. Before you insert an otoscope into someone's ear, bear in mind that a careful examiner never pokes any kind of instrument into a body orifice without watching to see where the instrument is going. Always look into the otoscope as you perform your inspection. Never penetrate deeper without first making absolutely certain that you have a clear and unobstructed path.

4. Now, with the otoscope light switched on, insert the tip of the funnel just inside the external auditory canal. Otoscopes come with an assortment of little funnels with various-sized ends for various-sized ear canals. Use the largest size funnel that will fit comfortably into the canal you are examining. If the funnel size is too small, it is very difficult to see anything at all.

5. Under direct observation, still pulling the ear flap backward, slowly insert the otoscope down the ear canal as far as it will comfortably and easily go, as long as you see nothing in the path ahead.

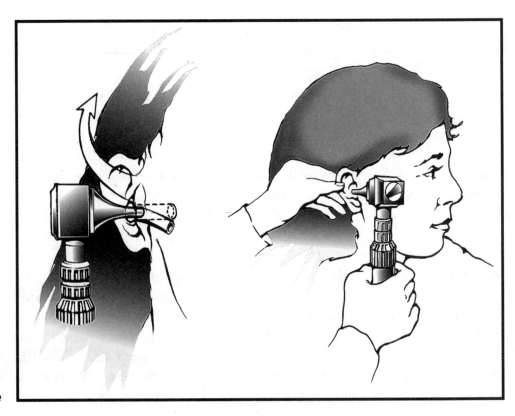

Using an Otoscope

Caution: It is important to look through the oto-scope as you insert it because there may be some wax or a foreign body such as a stone or a bean in the ear. By inserting the otoscope without watching, you could actually push this farther into the ear canal and do serious damage. It cannot be stressed too strongly that if you use an otoscope, you must watch where you are going.

6. The normal ear canal is a light tan color with just a blush of pink in it. You may also see a very dark, reddish-brown material about the consistency and color of very thick automobile grease. This is earwax and should be no cause for concern. Sometimes the wax only partially obstructs the canal and you can complete your examination by looking past it. You may find, however, that your view of the external auditory canal and the eardrum is entirely blocked by wax. If this is the case, you will have to remove it before you can complete your observations.

Removing Earwax

Earwax is easily removed by first softening the wax for several days with a drugstore preparation called Debrox®. Before you go ahead with this procedure, however, there is one very important precaution regarding the use of Debrox and the washing procedure that it involves. Sometimes as a result of a previous accident or infection, the eardrum has been ruptured, resulting in a permanent hole in the drum. You can see such a hole in the eardrum with your otoscope if wax does not obscure it. If you know or suspect that you have a hole in your eardrum, you should not use Debrox nor should you squirt water into your ear. Water can do permanent damage to the middle ear, so the ear-washing procedure that will be described should not be carried out if there is a hole in the eardrum.

Caution: If you don't know or if you aren't sure whether or not the eardrum is intact, ask your doctor before you squirt water into the ear.

1. Administer several drops of Debrox in the ear twice a day for two or three days.

2. You will find that the wax becomes so soft that it almost runs out. The ear can now be cleaned using an ear-cleaning syringe—a simple rubber squeeze bulb is quite adequate for this purpose. Before you proceed to rinse out the ear, look into it with your otoscope and make certain that the wax is soft and runny. If it still looks quite hard, give the Debrox another day or two to work.

3. To wash out the ear, fill the syringe with warm water and *gently* squirt the water into the ear canal. Place the pointed tip of the ear syringe very loosely into the canal.

Caution: You must not completely block the canal with the tip of the syringe or the water you are squirting in will have no place to go. You can do permanent harm to your ear by plugging the canal tightly with the tip of a rubber ear syringe and then squeezing hard.

4. With the tip of the syringe loosely inserted, the water will come running right back out, mixed with chunks of softened earwax.

Earwax is not the only material that may be found in the external auditory canal. Small foreign objects often find their way into the ear, especially in young children. Unless the foreign object you find is a piece of cotton that you can easily grab with a tweezers, do not attempt to remove it yourself. Specially designed tweezers are generally required for hard objects and attempts to remove a foreign object yourself will more often lead to accidentally pushing it farther in than actually retrieving it. It is very difficult to grasp a foreign object in the ear canal using conventional tweezers. Go to your doctor and have it done for you.

One other condition that you might conceivably find is a wet, greenish substance indicating an infection of the external auditory canal. This is invariably accompanied by great discomfort. An infection of the external auditory canal should be promptly treated with the appropriate antibiotic eardrops. Thus, if your initial inspection reveals a greenish, wet, messy-looking ear canal, you should visit your doctor without delay.

Inspecting the Eardrum

Once you have made certain that there is no earwax, no foreign body, and no infection present in the external auditory canal, you should be able to observe the eardrum using your otoscope.

1. Following the previous instructions regarding the use of an otoscope (reread the method for inspecting the external auditory canal in "Using an Otoscope"), straighten the ear canal by pulling the outer ear flap firmly backward and insert the otoscope down the ear canal as far as it will easily and comfortably go.

Caution: Remember to always look into the otoscope as you perform your inspection to make absolutely certain that you have a clear and unobstructed path.

2. If you have straightened the canal correctly, you should now be able to identify the eardrum. The eardrum, as you will recall, is a cone-shaped membrane stretched across the inner end of the external auditory canal. A common error in ear examinations is to mistake the canal wall for the drum. The walls of the external auditory canal and the eardrum are normally a dull, slightly pinkish tan. The eardrum, however, is a bit shiny compared with the canal wall and should reflect light back to you.

3. Under direct observation, move your otoscope around a bit both up and down and from side to side until you get a clear view of the drum. There is a small protrusion at one point where the middle-ear bones are attached on the inside.

This gives the eardrum the appearance of the top of a slightly rounded tent with the tent pole sticking up at you just a little.

Study the appearance of the eardrum carefully. An infection of the middle ear can affect the appearance of the eardrum in several ways. The mildest effect is simply a slight graying of color and a loss of the normal light reflection. Another form of middle-ear infection is indicated by a bluish eardrum. If an infection of the middle ear continues unchecked, the eardrum will become pink and eventually quite bright red. If an advanced middle-ear infection is present and the Eustachian tube is blocked, the eardrum may bulge considerably. A bulging, inflamed-looking eardrum indicates a severe infection of the middle ear. It will also be quite painful. If this goes unattended, the eardrum may rupture, resulting in substantial and sometimes permanent hearing loss. Should your examination reveal a bulging red drum or an eardrum with a gray or bluish cast, you should seek medical attention immediately.

After a middle-ear infection has been treated, the eardrum gradually returns to its normal, slightly rounded shape and recovers its slightly shiny surface. Sometimes a dark redness lingers around the edges of the drum as the infection clears up.

Even without an otoscope, it is possible to learn quite a bit about the ear simply by observing any discharge that comes out of the auditory canal. The wet, greenish substance that is characteristic of an external auditory canal infection usually comes running out at some point. With such infections the ear canal always feels painful or at least strange, and there is always some hearing loss on the affected side.

Earwax occasionally becomes fluid enough to run out of the ear, particularly at night if you sleep with your ear pressed against the pillow. The insulating qualities of the pillow warm up that side of your head just a bit, causing the wax to soften and run out of the ear. You may notice this on your pillow in the morning as a dry, crusted material and mistake it for blood. If you are unable to distinguish between earwax and dried blood, and you have reason to believe that your ear has bled, you should test the substance for traces of blood using the following test.

Testing for Bleeding from the Ear

Blood coming from the ear canal is a serious finding. It is never normal. There are a few very ordinary, unimportant reasons for ear bleeding such as pimples at the entrance to the canal, but in general the symptom is likely to be a serious one and should not be ignored. If you suspect that blood has come from your ear canal, you can quickly confirm your suspicions—or lay them to rest—using the same Hematest kit you use to test for blood in the stools (refer to Chapter 3 on the digestive process). The Hematest kit will detect traces of blood—if any are present—in a sample of material from the ear canal. You can purchase these kits in any well-stocked pharmacy.

1. The Hematest kit consists of a special filter paper and some hydrogen peroxide. Place a sample of the crusty dried material on the test paper.

2. Add the hydrogen peroxide according to the package instructions and observe the filter paper for a color change indicating the presence of blood. Blood will give a very strong, positive blue reaction. Earwax will give practically no color at all except for perhaps a little spreading of the brown tinge. A positive reaction from this test indicates bleeding from the ear canal, and you should consult your doctor without delay.

Hearing and Hearing Loss

Because the primary function of the ear is to hear, hearing testing is the best criterion of whether or not the ear is working properly. (A secondary function, balance, is dealt with in Chapter 6 on the nervous system.)

Human hearing is measured according to two scales. One scale tests your range of pitch—that is, the lowest and the highest tones that you can hear. This is measured in terms of cycles per second. Normal conversation registers about 1,000 cycles; a 6,000-cycle tone sounds like a very high squeak. Average human hearing ranges from a low of 20 to a high of 20,000 cycles per second. High-frequency hearing decreases with age, down to about 8,000 cycles per second for a fifty-year-old individual and 4,000 for an eighty-year-old. Rock-group musicians and their audiences whose ears have been assaulted by very loud music over a long period of time are especially vulnerable to high-frequency hearing loss.

A second scale—the decibel scale—measures human hearing in terms of intensity, or loudness. A whisper from four feet away measures about twenty decibels, and a normal conversation registers about sixty decibels.

Hearing is generally tested using an audiometer—a rather sophisticated piece of electronic equipment that measures both intensity of sound (loudness) and frequency (pitch). You cannot duplicate audiometer testing in your home, of course. It should be apparent from the preceding discussion, however, that we ordinarily use only a small part of our total hearing range, and that is the voice range. We are not commonly called on to discern very high, very low, or very soft sounds.

There are a number of observations you can make that may lead you to suspect that you or someone else in the family is suffering from a hearing deficiency:

- Seeming inattention when someone speaks
- Continually saying, "What?" or "Huh?"
- Difficulty hearing on the telephone
- Learning difficulties in school
- Problems in learning to speak
- Speaking considerably louder than seems necessary

Naturally, all of these may have other causes besides hearing loss, but any one of them should prompt you to consider a hearing test to be sure everything is all right. You can test your hearing at home in several ways to see if more extensive, professional testing is warranted.

Testing for Hearing Loss

Method 1. You will need a ticking watch or clock and a tape measure for this test. An easy method to quickly screen for hearing loss is to see how far away the ticking can be heard by a person known to have good hearing. Compare this with the farthest distance the *same* watch can be heard by the person being tested. Start at a distance where you are sure the watch is too far away to be heard and gradually bring it closer.

Method 2. Record a series of names and numbers on a tape recorder. Speak quietly, slowly, and distinctly, allowing enough time between items for a listener to write down the name or number. Keep your voice level; do not vary the volume.

Using headphones, the subject being tested plays the recording and writes down what he or she can hear. Listening with one ear at a time, gradually turn down the volume until the names and numbers no longer can be heard. Mark the spot on the volume control where the sound disappears. Compare the subject's ability to hear with that of someone known to have good hearing who takes the same test.

Method 3. You can also check for hearing loss using a tuning fork. A tuning fork rated at 256 cycles per second is commonly used. The cost of such an instrument is $10 to $15 at a medical-supply store, or you may find one you can borrow at a local high school physics laboratory.

A. Strike the tuning fork to make it vibrate.

B. Place the end of the stem of the fork against the skull behind the ear.

C. Ask the subject being tested to report when the sound can no longer be heard.

D. At this point, immediately bring the prongs of the fork to the subject's ear opening. If hearing is normal, a faint sound will again be heard by the subject.

E. Again, strike the tuning fork to make it vibrate.

F. Place the end of the stem on top of the subject's head at about the center.

G. If the sound is louder in one ear than in the other, this indicates some loss of hearing. (To understand this effect better, try it yourself and plug one ear at a time with your finger. The sound will become dramatically loud in the unplugged ear.)

The Nose

The average nose can identify about 4,000 different smells, and a trained nose can distinguish up to 10,000 different scents. If you were suddenly deprived of your vision and hearing, your nose would really come into its own, identifying people, houses, and even rooms by the sense of smell alone.

Investigators use their noses to solve all types of problems; your nose is the organ that warns when your pot roast is burning; your nose helps you enjoy the foods you like and reject those you don't like or that may not be good for you. On the other hand your nose can be a nuisance, getting in the way of kissing, dribbling when you would prefer it didn't, and never being quite the shape you want it to be to complement the rest of your face.

What you think of as your nose is actually two noses, one on either side of the septum—the partition of bone and cartilage that runs down the middle of the nasal cavity.

One of the primary functions of the nose is to clean and condition the air we breathe before it reaches the delicate tissues in the lungs. Long, coarse hairs just inside each nostril and the mucous membranes—spongy red tissue lining the nasal cavity—filter out dust and other contaminants and help warm and humidify cold, dry air. This latter function is assisted greatly by the nasal turbinates. These are three little chips of bone, the biggest about an inch long, that protrude from the upper septum in each nostril. The nasal turbinates are also covered by mucous membrane. When you breathe in cold air, this tissue swells with blood, providing a greater surface area for warming the frigid air.

The other function of the nose, of course, is smell. The olfactory area of your nose is contained in a surprisingly small patch of tissue about the size of a postage stamp, yellow-brown in color, located in the roof of each nostril.

Finally, the nasal chamber also includes eight sinus cavities. These are hollow pockets in the surrounding bone lined with the same mucous membrane found in the nasal passages. While the sinus cavities serve to lighten the skull (solid bone would add considerably to the weight of the skull) and add resonance to our voice, they are often troublesome. The sinuses communicate with the rest of the nasal cavity via narrow channels that are easily infected. When this happens, the opening into the main chamber becomes swollen and closes, and pressure builds up within the sinus cavity, causing considerable pain and discomfort. This inflammation of the mucous membrane lining these airspaces is called sinusitis. Because the sinuses are enclosed by bone, you will not be able to observe them in your examination of the nose.

Observing the External Nose

An external examination of the nose involves a critical look at its shape, color, and configuration.

The nose is normally bilaterally symmetric—that is, one side should look much like the other—and the midline, or bridge, should be straight. If the midline of the nose is shifted markedly to one side, this is an indication of an abnormality, usually the result of a trauma or accident.

A bulbous, red nose is definitely abnormal but, contrary to popular belief, it is not necessarily an indication of alcoholism. A condition called acne rosacea, caused by excessive flushing of the blood vessels in the nose and cheek, also causes a red nose, and so do certain vitamin deficiencies and infections. A general enlargement of the tissues of the nose can also occur. Several types of disorders can cause this, most of which are fairly rare. So if your nose has taken on a red, bulbous appearance or seems larger than normal, you should bring these findings to the attention of your doctor.

Examining the Inside of the Nose

An internal examination of the nose can be carried out using either a penlight or a nasal speculum. If you have purchased an otoscope, you probably already have a nasal speculum. This is the largest of the little funnels that come with the otoscope. Somewhat shorter and fatter than the rest, it is specially designed for looking into the nose. If you don't have one of these, you can do almost as well by looking into the nose with just a penlight.

1. Press the tip of the nose inward to widen the openings and peer upward into the nasal cavity. If you are using a nasal speculum, you must take the same care you took when inspecting the ear. That means never insert the instrument up the nostril without looking where you are going. Check to make sure that there are no foreign objects that could be pushed farther into the nasal cavity by your speculum. As with the ear, if a foreign object is lodged fairly far into the nose, special instruments are required to retrieve it and this should not be attempted at home.

2. Examine the mucous membrane that lines the inside of the nose. This is normally pinkish in color and is covered with a number of fine hairs. When you come down with a cold, this lining becomes swollen and reddened. The nose feels stuffy, and a watery discharge is present. As the cold wears on, this discharge becomes somewhat thickened and yellow. The mucous membrane also becomes swollen during an allergic nasal reaction such as hay fever, but in this case, the swollen membrane is rather pale in color and the discharge, while profuse, is quite watery.

3. Inspect the central nasal septum. This is the wall between the two nostrils. The septum should be straight and smooth, its mucous membrane pinkish. A hole in the septum is not normal. Should you discover a perforation, you should seek medical advice promptly.

4. Locate the nasal turbinates. Higher up in the nasal cavity, on either side of the septum, are three small, shelflike protrusions. These are the nasal turbinates and they, too, are covered with the same mucous membrane that lines the rest of the cavity. You may not be able to see the turbinates without a nasal speculum.

5. Look for polyps. These are boggy, swollen, saclike masses that can block air passages and sinus channels. They resemble little mushrooms and may be quite small or as large as a grape. Polyps are often found in conjunction with allergies. These should be reported to a physician.

Your examination of the nose should conclude with a test of your ability to perceive different odors. Our sense of smell is controlled by the olfactory nerve, which is the first cranial nerve. A test of first cranial nerve function can be found in Chapter 6, titled "How to Test Your Nervous System."

The Mouth

The mouth is an easy subject for self-examination simply because it is so conveniently situated and because abnormalities are so readily apparent once you know what you're looking for. You can diagnose a number of abnormal conditions and get a good look inside this vital cavity with the aid of a few simple tools. You will need a penlight, a wooden tongue blade, and a dental mirror. You can purchase an inexpensive plastic dental mirror and tongue blades at most drugstores. The handle of a teaspoon may be used in place of a tongue blade.

Inspecting the Tongue

A good place to start your inspection of the mouth is with the tongue. The tongue is a complex assortment of muscles and nerves enclosed in mucous membrane. The mucous membrane covering is studded with taste buds on both the top and bottom surfaces. These taste buds transmit sour, bitter, sweet, and salty taste sensations to the brain via special nerves. You can test your sense of taste by checking this aspect of seventh and ninth cranial nerve function with the tests found in Chapter 6 on testing the nervous system.

Another cranial nerve, the twelfth, controls the muscles of the tongue; this, too, is tested with the nervous system. In addition to detecting taste sensations, the tongue is an invaluable aid in preparing food for the digestive process and in forming speech sounds.

You can get the best view of your tongue by grasping the tip with a small, 4 × 4-inch piece of clean cloth and gently pulling it into view in front of your bathroom mirror. Rub warm water over the mirror to prevent it from fogging up when you breathe on it.

1. Inspect the size, shape, and color of your tongue. The shape of the tongue may vary from one person to another; some tongues are flat and pointed while others are fuller and more rounded. The surface of the tongue should be pink and somewhat rough. Observe the coating on top of the tongue. It is normally a whitish-gray color that may be more noticeable on some days than others. Smokers typically have a heavier coating on their tongues, particularly in the morning after they get up. A greenish-white fungus sometimes appears on the surface of the tongue, and if you have been taking antibiotics, your tongue may have a black coating. But neither these nor most other discolorations of a normally rough tongue are of serious consequence. A smooth, beefy-red tongue, however, is abnormal and occurs in several diseases. If your tongue feels too big for your mouth or seems to have shrunk and you have not recently either lost teeth or acquired dentures, you should bring this to the attention of your doctor.

2. Identify the taste buds. Blot your tongue dry with a paper towel and observe it closely using your penlight. You should be able to see the taste buds. They look a bit like bunches of tiny strings or soft, miniature brushes. As mentioned previously, the sensation of taste is controlled by cranial nerves, which are tested in Chapter 6.

3. Look for sores. Observe all surfaces of the tongue for lumps, open sores, ulcers, swellings, pain, or tenderness. None of these conditions are normal and any that persist for longer than a week should receive medical attention.

Checking the Salivary Ducts

Your mouth also contains salivary glands, vital glands that are often overlooked and unappreciated. There are three of them, actually, one in each cheek and one under the tongue. The saliva produced by these glands lubricates your food, aids in swallowing food and digesting it, and plays a role in fighting tooth decay by neutralizing acid in the mouth. You should be able to locate your salivary glands and observe them in action.

1. Holding your cheek out a bit with your fingers, run your tongue blade along the inside of your cheek. This will tend to exaggerate any bumps. You should notice a little pimplelike bump in the middle of the cheek, opposite the last two upper teeth. This is the outlet of a salivary duct, from which saliva is introduced into the mouth. You will find one on each cheek. A third duct is located under the tongue, directly behind the lower front teeth.

2. You can observe the function of the salivary ducts with this simple test. Do not eat, drink, or chew gum for a few hours. This lulls the salivary glands into a resting state. Then chew on a sugared slice of lemon for about five seconds or so. Now look at the salivary gland outlets again and you should be able to see saliva pouring from the ducts.

3. Check all three ducts. The outlets do occasionally get plugged up. In such cases the saliva backs up in the duct and the gland swells. This can become very painful; if it happens, you should see your doctor at once.

Inspecting Your Teeth

A thorough inspection of your teeth can reveal a variety of potentially troublesome conditions including cavities, unnatural gaps, the presence of plaque, improper bite, tooth sensitivity, stains, and nerve damage.

Before beginning your inspection, brush your teeth and then rinse thoroughly with lukewarm water. Run warm water over your dental mirror to keep it from fogging up during your examination.

If a tooth is bothering you or you find something suspicious, you want to be able to describe the location of the tooth to your dentist. And when you record in your health record what work was performed after a visit

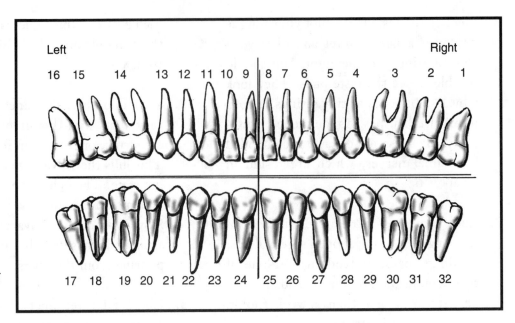

A Numbering System for Your Teeth

to the dentist, you should be able to describe the exact location of the teeth that were worked on.

The accompanying illustration of a full complement of teeth is numbered as most dentists number them, the top right tooth being number one and the bottom right tooth being number thirty-two. Identify your teeth according to these numbers even if some are missing. In addition to numbering, dentists refer to the lingual side of the tooth—the inside facing the tongue— and the facial side—the part of the tooth facing your lips.

Checking for Cavities

Cavities are most commonly found in three areas: between the teeth, at the gum line, and in the grooves on the tops of the teeth. A cavity is indicated by a small hole, usually stained by a blackish color. (The hole on the

outside, by the way, is very much smaller than the hole being made on the inside.)

1. Examine each tooth in your mouth carefully and methodically for evidence of decay. You may prefer to work with a partner and inspect each other's teeth. To view all surfaces of your teeth, you will have to use your penlight in coordination with your dental mirror. To do this, hold your dental mirror behind the tooth surface that you wish to observe, shine the penlight into the mirror and let it reflect its light onto the tooth. In this way, the mirror serves to bend the light directly onto a hidden surface. Use your mirror to help keep your tongue out of the way. All of this takes some coordination, but you should be able to master the technique with a bit of practice.

2. Be sure not to miss any tooth surface in your examination. If you find a suspicious

spot, make a note of it and report it to your dentist.

Examining Unnatural Gaps

The normal complement of adult teeth is thirty-two. This includes your four wisdom teeth that you may have had taken out, or that may be hidden in the gum. Starting with the tooth farthest back in your upper right jaw, count your teeth. You will need to use your dental mirror to do this; don't go by touch alone. If you have fewer than twenty-eight teeth, you should carefully examine the gaps where teeth are missing.

Where a tooth is missing, check the corresponding tooth in the other jaw to see if it is growing into the void left by the missing tooth. To do this, close your jaws and then separate your lips with your fingers; look at the tooth opposite the empty space to see if it extends down (or up) farther than the teeth on either side of it. If you find this to be so, you should bring it to the attention of your dentist without delay. If any of your teeth have begun to move or grow into a space where a tooth is missing, this, too, is a serious finding that requires professional attention.

Testing for Plaque

Plaque is a sticky, almost invisible film composed of bacteria, saliva, and food debris that clings to tooth surfaces, eventually causing tooth decay and gum disease. You can check your teeth for evidence of plaque by using disclosing tablets. These tablets, available at most drugstores in the toothbrush section, contain a harmless dye that will turn plaque bright red so you can locate and remove it more effectively. Do not be concerned about the tablet staining the inside of your mouth; the color will disappear within a few hours.

1. After cleaning your teeth, chew a disclosing tablet well, let it dissolve in your saliva, and swish it around in your mouth; then empty your mouth.

2. Examine your teeth using your penlight and dental mirror as described earlier so that you can observe both the inner and outer surfaces. The red-stained areas represent deposits of plaque that can be removed with more thorough brushing and flossing.

Testing for Malocclusion

An improper bite, called malocclusion, is one in which the teeth do not come together uniformly and evenly. Many of us have some degree of malocclusion; a common form is jaw-to-jaw mismatch in which either the upper or the lower jaw protrudes. Malocclusion can also result from crooked teeth and from high fillings. A high filling, as the name implies, is slightly higher than the teeth on either side. Thus when you bite, you will be hitting first on this spot. Continually impacting on a high spot when you chew, in addition to being uncomfortable, can damage a tooth.

A high spot can easily be detected by closing your teeth together gently. Rub your teeth together from side to side. If there is a high spot, you will feel it. Should you find such a spot you should bring it to the attention of your dentist. Your dentist is usually very careful to check for a high spot when he or she completes a new filling. Don't be afraid to report that you feel a high spot when the dentist asks.

Testing for Tooth Sensitivity

1. Healthy teeth should not be particularly sensitive to pressure, heat, or cold. If you have reason to believe that a particular tooth is unsound, gently tap its upper surface with a spoon handle. If it hurts or is even moderately sensitive, there is probably something wrong with the tooth. A normal tooth does not hurt when you tap it with a spoon handle. If there is a question in your mind concerning the response of a particular tooth, tap the same tooth on the other side of the jaw for comparison.

2. Next, swish some hot water and then cold water around in your mouth. Neither of these should cause you any undue discomfort. Once in a while your teeth may react to extreme temperatures, but persistent temperature sensitivity in one or more teeth is not normal and should be brought to the attention of your dentist.

Because the mouth, ears, and nose are so closely related, pain in one place may be referred to another nearby. Tooth pain may be felt in your ear, or a sinus problem may be referred to your upper teeth. It is not smart, however, to ignore tooth pain from whatever source or to attempt to cover it up with medications. If tooth pain is mild, you might want to wait a day or two to see if it goes away by itself. But if pain persists or increases in intensity, see your dentist at once; an abscess could be forming.

Diagnosing Nerve Damage in a Tooth

Stains on the teeth can be yellow, orange, brown, red, and even green. Most of them are harmless (as long as they are not hiding evidence of decay) and can be removed with a professional cleaning. You should be concerned, however, about dark stains in a tooth that was recently white and healthy looking, because this may indicate damage to the nerve root.

A discoloration in just one tooth or in two adjacent teeth that were white and healthy looking a short time ago should be viewed with suspicion, particularly if you recently received a blow to the mouth. (Note: Children commonly get struck in the mouth in the course of play and may not recall the incident several days later.) A blow to the mouth does not have to be powerful to kill the nerve in a tooth, just well placed.

If the nerve root is damaged, the tooth begins to die, changing color in the process. This color change can range from gray to yellow to brown or black. If you notice this kind of localized discoloration in a recently healthy tooth, you should treat it as a dental emergency.

Checking for Signs of Gum Disease

An inspection of your teeth is not complete without a close examination of your gums. Normal, healthy gums have five characteristics:

1. They are firm and fit snugly around each tooth.

2. They are pink to dark pink in color or even whitish-pink. An inflamed red appearance is abnormal.

3. Gum tissue forms a "V" between the teeth.

4. Gums have little dotlike indentations, called stippling, especially in the areas closest to the teeth.

5. Gum tissue forms tiny "collars" around the base of each tooth.

To identify these last two characteristics, you will need to blot dry a section of gum tissue and observe it closely using your penlight.

Gum disease can take many forms and is an insidious process that leads, if unchecked, to substantial tooth loss. You can spot gum disease at an early stage, when it is still treatable, by performing the following inspection at frequent intervals.

Keeping in mind how normal, healthy gums look, examine your gums for the five characteristics previously described. Use your dental mirror and penlight to examine hard-to-see areas of gum tissue. As you perform your inspection, check for these telltale signs of gum disease.

1. Bleeding gums. Healthy gums do not bleed. If your gums bleed during brushing or while eating, they are not normal. If you are not sure if your gums bleed or not, gently run a length of dental floss between two teeth and against the area of gum in question. If this procedure causes the gum to bleed, this is an abnormal finding that probably indicates some degree of gum disease.

2. Pus in gums. A white, puslike substance exuding from the tip of the gums is abnormal. If the tip of the gum between the teeth looks white and pus-filled, put your finger on the gum and press inward and upward. Traces of pus or blood as a result of this procedure are abnormal.

3. Receding gums. The gums should appear to be attached to the enamel, or white part, of the tooth. If the gum appears to be receding from the tooth, thus exposing more of the tooth and even the root to view, this should be brought to the attention of your dentist without delay.

4. Swollen, puffy, red gums. Gums that are angry or inflamed-looking are unhealthy. Check closely around the base of each tooth for this abnormal reddening.

5. Painful, burning gums. Gums that are tender to the touch and have a stinging, burning sensation are probably diseased.

Gum disease is also likely to be accompanied by bad breath and, in advanced cases, a slight fever as well. Never underestimate the role of a healthy mouth in your general well-being. It is a mistake to assume that a toothache or gum disease is of minor consequence. Like any threat to your system, either can draw on the body's resources to mobilize an attack against the invading infection; this is a debilitating process that saps your vitality. If the infection continues unchecked, your teeth will be only the first casualty in what can be a long, miserable war.

Examining the Throat and Tonsils

Examining the throat requires working with a partner. The landmarks of the throat can be identified rather easily using a penlight and a tongue depressor. (The handle of a spoon may be substituted for a wooden tongue blade.)

Ask your partner to open his or her mouth wide and relax the tongue. In many people you will be able to see the throat clearly without the aid of a tongue depressor. If you have trouble seeing past the tongue, place the tongue blade or spoon handle on the surface of the tongue about two-thirds of the way back and press down gently. You must be gentle but firm when doing this and position the tongue blade carefully. If it is placed too far back on the tongue, you are likely to gag your subject and not see anything. If your tongue blade is too far forward, you will not be able to press down enough of the tongue to improve your view of the throat.

Shine your flashlight into the mouth. (If you purchased an otoscope for examining the ear, check to see if your otoscope head converts into a throat illuminator.) With the tongue out of the way, you should be able to see the throat clearly. The wall at the very rear of the mouth belongs to a tube called the pharynx, which connects the nasal cavity with the oral cavity and continues on down to the esophagus and, eventually, the stomach.

One obvious landmark here is a little tongue of tissue that hangs down from the roof of the mouth to the center of the throat. This is not, as many people mistakenly believe, a tonsil. This is the uvula, and every time you swallow it acts as a flap, closing off the passage to the nasal cavity and thus ensuring that your meal goes down the pharynx instead of up your nose. Your tonsils are located on either side of the uvula, behind little curtains of tissue. These little curtains on each side of the rear wall of the mouth are called the tonsillar pillars. The tonsils protrude out a bit from behind the tonsillar pillars, one on either side.

1. Using your flashlight and tongue blade in the procedure previously described, locate the tonsils and the tonsillar pillars.

2. Like the membranes inside the nose and mouth, the tonsillar pillars and the tonsils should be uniformly pinkish in color. The tonsils are normally about the size of a cherry, and the surface is covered with a series of irregular, barely visible grooves. Healthy tonsils are often almost completely hidden behind the tonsillar pillars.

3. When the throat becomes infected, the tonsils enlarge dramatically, particularly in children, and all the tissues of the throat become red and inflamed.

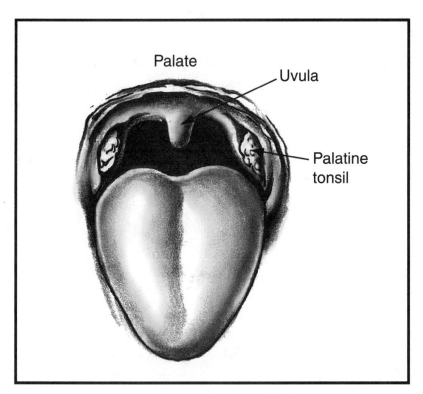

Palate

Uvula

Palatine
tonsil

Position of the Tonsils

4. Infected tonsils may also show patches of white material in the normal cracks and grooves on the surface. White patches on the tonsils are characteristic of streptococcal infections, known as strep throat, and are therefore an important finding. Anyone who has a fever, a sore throat, swollen lymph nodes at the angle of the jaw and along the front of the neck, and enlarged tonsils with patches of white should see his or her doctor promptly.

People with a streptococcal infection in their throat usually feel quite sick. If left untreated, particularly in children, a streptococcal infection can lead to far more serious problems than a sore throat. Scarlet fever, for one, is actually a gener-alized streptococcal infection that has spread through the whole body. One of the most serious types of valvular heart disease is caused by a streptococcal infection of the heart following a strep throat. Uncontrolled, this can cause extensive damage that will eventually require open-heart surgery. The kidneys, too, are a potential target for the streptococcal bacteria. It is primarily with the hope of avoiding these life-threatening aftereffects that physicians are so anxious to treat streptococcal infections. It is an easy disease to treat, as the vast majority of strains of the bacteria are presently sensitive to penicillin, although some have become penicillin-resistant over the years. If you suspect you have strep throat, you should immediately consult a doctor.

6

How to Test Your Nervous System

The nervous system, consisting of the brain, the spinal cord, and nerves that stream out to every part of the body is unquestionably the most awesome structure of the human body. The central nervous system functions as the body's command headquarters, processing incoming information, controlling body functions, and making decisions at a rate that would blow a fuse on the most sophisticated computer.

Despite its staggering complexity, a basic evaluation of the nervous system is carried out using very simple equipment. Some tests are carried out by observation alone. Some require a simple hat pin, some a flashlight, and some a little rubber hammer. Unlike other medical specialists, neurologists rely less on x-rays, complicated tests, and elaborate equipment than on close observation and careful reasoning. The blink of an eye— or the absence of a blink—is worth a thousand x-rays to the neurologist. The simplest reflex response tells a skilled specialist volumes about the subject's nerve pathways.

Obviously, it takes years of training and experience to detect subtle symptoms of neurological disorders and interpret their significance. Still, it is possible to perform a fairly comprehensive evaluation of the nervous system through self-testing. The simple tests and observations described later on in this chapter should help you spot potentially troublesome abnormalities that should be brought to the attention of a specialist, and they will also tell you when things are normal and working well. First, however, a brief review of the anatomy of the nervous system will give you a better understanding of the tests that follow.

The Brain

Of all the organs in the body, the brain is the last to give up its secrets. Like outer space, the brain is one of the "last frontiers" left to penetrate. Many aspects of brain function are not at all understood, and there is a growing body of evidence that the brain is more than a supercomplicated computer made up of nerve cells and connecting elements. Recent findings suggest that the brain probably also secretes a number of subtle, hormonelike substances that tell the master endocrine gland—the pituitary—what to do.

Microscopically, the brain consists of about 30 billion neurons, or nerve cells, supported by a fine network of glial cells, plus a wealth of blood vessels to provide nourishment for the cells.

Two great lobes of the brain, called the cerebral hemispheres, lie adjacent to each other and fill most of the skull. Deep inside these cerebral hemispheres is an open space filled with a watery substance called cerebral spinal fluid. This fluid fills the hollow spaces in the brain called the ventricles and also the space surrounding the spinal cord. If a doctor does a procedure called a spinal tap, he or she is taking a small sample of this fluid for analysis.

The cerebral hemispheres control virtually all the higher functions, including reason, speech, memory, smell, taste, vision, and movement. One hemisphere is always dominant over the other. If you are right-handed, your left hemisphere is probably dominant; if you are left-handed, your right hemisphere is likely the dominant one. The dominant hemisphere usually controls speech. This and other general areas of the brain that control certain functions have been well established. For example, the sense of smell is located near the front of the cerebral hemispheres, and the sense of vision near the back. Muscle control is located along the sides.

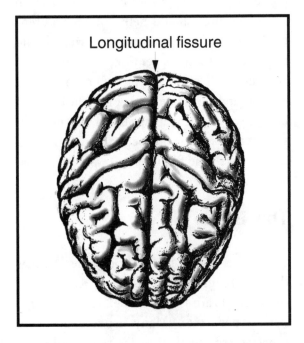

The Brain, Top View

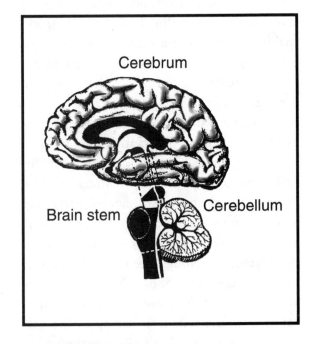

The Brain, Side View

The next major segment of the brain, called the cerebellum, sits beneath and toward the rear half of the great cerebral hemispheres and is also divided into two sections. The cerebellum controls functions you are generally unaware of, such as balance and kinesthesia. Kinesthesia is the ability to know where a part of your body is located without looking at it. That is to say, you know that your arm is hanging down at your side or pointing up in the air without looking at it. You know this because you have kinesthetic sense.

The final part of the brain is the brain stem. This is actually the upper end of the spinal cord and is shaped like the rounded knob on the end of a straight-handled cane. The brain stem goes up just in front of the cerebellum and tucks up underneath and into the cerebral hemispheres. The brain stem controls what are referred to as vegetative functions. These include, among others, breathing and heartbeat, which continue whether you are awake or asleep, aware of them or not aware of them.

If part of the brain is destroyed, some body function usually disappears. For example, when someone has a stroke, the blood supply to part of one of the cerebral hemispheres is usually cut off. This means that the part of the brain nourished by that particular blood vessel dies from lack of oxygen. It does this in very short order—usually no more than five minutes without oxygen is enough to destroy brain cells. And once they are gone, they are gone for good. There is no regrowth. The brain may learn to adapt or get along without certain cells by setting up compensating networks of nerve connections, but there is no growth of new brain cells after an injury.

The Spinal Cord

Continuing down from the brain stem is the spinal cord, which is housed in and protected by the bony spinal column. The spinal cord is sometimes thought of as simply a cable, or trunk line, of nerve fibers connecting the brain with the rest of the body, but it is actually much more than this. The spinal cord carries out some functions that might ordinarily be thought of as brain functions. For example, the simple reflex arc is actually a spinal-cord function. If you tap someone's knee in the right place, the leg jerks. It's not the brain telling the leg to jerk, however, but the spinal cord. This simple knee-jerk reaction is called an arc because the nerves that receive the tap from the hammer send the signal to the spinal cord; the signal is processed right there, and the message directing the muscle to jerk is sent right back. You don't need your brain to jerk your knee when it is tapped.

The Peripheral Nerves

The final element of the nervous system, after the brain and the spinal cord, consists of the peripheral nerves that run uninterrupted from connections in the spinal cord to all parts of your body. Thirty-one pairs of nerve bundles branch out from the spinal cord. Almost half are sensory nerves that convey information *to* the brain; the rest are motor nerves that transmit orders *from* the brain to the muscles. These are the final functioning messengers in the nervous system. More than any other part of the nervous system, the peripheral nerves can be thought of as a network of wires that connect the various organs and extremities of the body with the brain.

There is never just a single nerve connecting the spinal cord to a limb, however; there are many, many of them. Each small, special part of the muscle has its own nerve. What anatomists and surgeons often refer to as a single nerve, such as the large radial nerve in the arm, is not a single nerve at all but a bundle of nerves. If the entire bundle is interrupted, those fingers that it controls will hang limply and not work at all. If the bundle is cut only partway through, certain functions of some of the fingers will probably remain. It all depends on which of the nerves inside the bundle are interrupted.

Testing the Cranial Nerves

When a neurologist examines your nervous system, he or she usually begins with a special set of nerves called the cranial nerves. These are special nerves because, instead of coming off the spinal cord as all other major nerves do, the cranial nerves emanate directly from the base of the brain. There are twelve pairs of cranial nerves, with one nerve of each pair for the right side of the body and one for the left.

Because nerves branching off some cranial nerves serve different organs, a single cranial nerve may control several body functions. Testing for one function does not mean that the total nerve bundle is in good working order. And because muscles and nerves are so closely related in their functioning, it is often difficult to know when a

dysfunction is the fault of a muscle or a nerve. So while the following tests are interesting and informative, it should be kept in mind that they are not of themselves conclusive. Whenever some lack of function or abnormal functioning of a body part or organ is noticed, it should, of course, be called to a doctor's attention.

Following are a series of tests you can use to check the functioning of the cranial nerves.

Testing the Olfactory Nerve

1. The olfactory nerve controls your sense of smell. Assemble an assortment of small bottles of flavor extracts, the kind you find in the spice section of the supermarket. Use these: vanilla, peppermint, almond, and cherry.

2. Cover the bottles so that only the mouth of the jar is exposed.

3. Smell each of them. If you can identify all four scents correctly, the olfactory nerve is said to be intact and functioning.

Testing the Optic Nerve and Nerves That Control Eye Movement

The visual acuity tests and field of vision tests described in Chapter 4 will tell you if your optic nerve is intact. If you can see, it's OK. To check the nerves that control eye movements, do the following:

1. The person being tested should stare intently at a small object, such as the tip of a pencil.

2. Direct your subject to follow the pencil with his or her eyes only—the head should remain still. Move the pencil from side to side and up and down, and notice how the eyes move to follow it.

3. The eyes should move fully and in coordination with each other.

If double vision should suddenly occur during this test, it may indicate some degree of malfunction of one of the muscles that moves the eyes. It is often difficult to determine if one or more nerves is at fault or if it is a muscle weakness, without sophisticated testing by an ophthalmologist.

Testing the Oculomotor Nerve

The oculomotor nerve is one of several serving the motor functions of the eyes that can be tested separately from those just described because it controls the opening and closing of the eye's pupil.

1. Shine a flashlight into one eye and then the other. Shine it from the side rather than directly into the eye; a second or two is enough.

2. The pupils of *both* eyes should constrict in response to light shined into either eye.

3. If the pupil remains dilated and unresponsive to light, a problem with the oculomotor nerve is a possibility.

As noted in Chapter 4, drugs and certain illnesses or injuries can also affect the pupil-

lary reflex. But if this reflex is missing for any reason, you want to see a doctor and find out why.

Testing for Light-Touch Sensation

The trigeminal nerve, sometimes called the trifacial, is the chief sensory nerve of the face and head. Here is a simple way to test it:

1. Have the person being tested close his or her eyes.

2. Touch the face at different points with a wisp of cotton. Ask your subject to report when the touch is felt.

3. An inability to sense two or more touches is considered an abnormal finding.

(The trigeminal also controls sensation over the white part of your eye that makes you blink when the eyeball is touched.)

4. Twist the wisp of cotton to a point.

5. Have the subject stare straight ahead at some object.

6. Bring the wisp of cotton in toward the eye from the very outer edge. Make sure the subject is staring intently straight ahead so as not to see the cotton coming.

7. If the eye blinks when the cotton is touched to the white of the eye, the trigeminal nerve is normal.

If the trigeminal is impaired, the person will not feel the cotton against the eye that is touched and the blink response will not occur in *either* eye. If, on the other hand, the eyelid of the *opposite* eye closes when one eye is touched, a lesion or impairment of a *facial* nerve is suspected.

Testing the Facial Nerve and Taste Sensation

Among other things, the facial nerve controls taste sensation in the front two-thirds of the tongue. Just as every shade in the rainbow is based on some combination of the three primary colors—red, yellow, and blue—so, too, are the countless tastes that we enjoy composed of a mingling of four primary tastes—salt, sour, sweet, and bitter. Thus, you can check this aspect of seventh-nerve function by distinguishing among these four primary tastes:

1. Prepare separate solutions of each of the four primary taste sensations in little cups: a strong solution of ordinary sugar in water, a strong solution of ordinary table salt in water, a concentrated solution of instant coffee (one teaspoon of instant coffee in two tablespoons of hot water), and either lemon juice or vinegar. Rinse your mouth with water before beginning the test and between testing each of the four primary tastes.

2. Take a cotton-tipped swab, dip it in one of the solutions and touch it to one side of your tongue fairly far forward

but not at the very tip. (Note: When doing this test, it is important to place a very small amount of the fluid well to one side of the midline of the tongue. If a trace of fluid seeps across to the other side, you will not have a reliable test because you may actually be tasting the solution with the other side of your tongue.)

3. Test each of the four taste sensations on one side of the tongue, and then repeat and test on the other side. You should be able to taste each solution correctly and separately on each side of your tongue. If you cannot distinguish between any two of them, you may have a problem with the facial nerve.

The Facial Nerve and Bell's Palsy

Bell's palsy is a sudden onset of facial paralysis that can happen at any age. There is a flattening of the muscles of one side of the face, a crooked smile, and one eye appears to be opened wider than the other or may not be able to be closed at all. Speech becomes difficult.

It is easy to confuse Bell's palsy with a stroke. The difference is that Bell's palsy affects only the face muscles and not the arms or legs. It is a malfunctioning of the facial nerve, but no one knows for sure what causes it or how to cure it. Treatment is usually palliative—whatever makes the symptoms and the patient feel better. The good news is that for the vast majority of those afflicted, recovery is complete or nearly complete.

Testing the Auditory Nerve

The auditory nerve has two functions. One function is hearing: If your hearing is adequate, then that aspect of the auditory nerve function is normal. Part of the auditory nerve also leads to the semicircular canals in the inner ear, which affect balance and position sense. While balance and position sense are also assisted by feedback from the muscle system, you can get a pretty accurate assessment of this aspect of auditory nerve function with the following simple test:

1. Stand with your feet together, your eyes closed, and your arms down at your sides. Direct a partner to give you a sudden, gentle push backward, forward, or to one side, but not so hard as to knock you over.

2. If you have a normal balance mechanism, your partner will not have to catch you to prevent you from falling; instead, you will immediately correct for the unexpected shove. Disorders of this function of the auditory nerve may also have associated feelings of dizziness and some degree of hearing loss.

Disorders of the last four cranial nerves are harder to pinpoint because their individual functions are difficult to isolate. For instance, the ninth cranial nerve, called the glossopharyngeal nerve, controls a number of functions that are shared by two other cranial nerves. Within this network of shared functions, however, there are also some functions that are controlled individually by the last four cranial nerves. These lend themselves nicely to home testing and provide a basic assessment of each of these nerves.

Testing the Glossopharyngeal Nerve

The ninth cranial nerve regulates two functions of its own—one is taste on the back third of the tongue, and the other is sensation in the back of the throat. A test of this nerve is just like the taste test described earlier for the front part of the tongue.

1. Use the same four solutions you prepared to test taste on the front two-thirds of the tongue—concentrated solutions of sugar, salt, instant coffee, and lemon or vinegar.

2. Using a cotton-tipped swab, place the drops of solution on the rear third of the tongue. Be sure you test far enough back. Test both sides of the tongue, being careful not to test too close to the midline. You should be able to taste each solution separately and correctly on each side of the rear third of your tongue. If you cannot distinguish between any two of them, you may have a problem with the ninth cranial nerve.

Testing Sensation in the Throat— the Vagus Nerve

Stroking the back of the throat normally produces gagging. The presence of a gag reflex is one indication that the tenth cranial nerve, called the vagus, is functioning. The vagus nerve participates in a great many internal functions. Parts of the vagus extend all the way down to the stomach and are involved in the secretion of stomach acid. Other branches of this nerve control some of the muscles in the palate that help form normal speech sounds. If, over a period of weeks or months, your speech develops a slightly nasal quality that you are unable to control, this may be a sign of a problem with the vagus nerve. If indeed this is happening, the uvula should deviate to one side. The uvula is the little tongue of tissue that hangs down from the back of the palate, or roof, of the mouth. If there is a nasal quality to the speech and the uvula deviates to one side, this suggests a vagus-nerve disorder.

To test for sensation on the back wall of the pharynx, or throat, you will need a thin straw with a bit of cotton attached to one end.

1. Open your mouth wide and have your partner *gently* rub the wisp of cotton against the back of your throat.

2. To get your tongue out of the way, say "aah." Be sure your partner does not poke too hard; a light touch is all that is needed to determine if there is sensation in this area.

3. Some people have a very active gag reflex and will be made extremely uncomfortable by the lightest touch. Others will be able to tolerate some stroking. Both responses are normal. An absence of response, however, is not normal and may indicate vagus-nerve malfunction.

Testing the Spinal Accessory Nerve

The eleventh cranial nerve, referred to as the spinal accessory nerve, controls certain muscles in the shoulders. You can easily check this aspect of eleventh-nerve function by asking your partner to help you perform the following test.

1. Raise both your shoulders as if shrugging them, but instead of lowering them, hold them elevated.

2. Have your partner push down hard on both shoulders at the same time, exerting an equal amount of force on both sides.

3. If one shoulder can be pushed down with relative ease while the other still offers good resistance, there may be some impairment of the eleventh cranial nerve.

Testing the Hypoglossal Nerve

To test the twelfth cranial nerve, called the hypoglossal (from *hypo* = under and *glossa* = tongue), look into a mirror and stick your tongue out. Normally, your tongue protrudes straight out, though a slight deviation to one side is not uncommon. If, however, your tongue protrudes crookedly to one side of the mouth or the other, this suggests a lesion of one side of the twelfth cranial nerve. When *both* sides of this nerve are affected, it is difficult to stick out the tongue at all. In either case, you would probably notice a clumsiness of the tongue that would show up in your speech.

Testing the Spinal Nerves

In addition to the twelve pairs of cranial nerves that stem directly from the base of the brain, thirty-one pairs of nerves branch off from the spinal cord to various parts of the body. Unlike the cranial nerves that we evaluated one by one, these spinal nerves, as they are called, are initially tested as a system according to three broad areas of function: sensory functioning, motor functioning, and mental functioning. You can make a good general assessment of your own nervous system by performing the following tests, which check these three functions. Defects revealed by any of these tests should be brought to the attention of a neurologist for more in-depth examination.

How to Test Sensory Functioning

Sensory input provides the nervous system with a wealth of information that enables us to distinguish between sandpaper and silk or hot and cold, to "see" the shape of an object by touch alone, and to know where our hands and feet are and what they are up to even when we can't see them. This kind of information constitutes our most basic link with the world around us.

Simply stated, it works like this: Special sensing or sensory cells near the surface of the skin detect sensations of touch such as hot or cold, firm pressure or light pressure, smoothness or roughness, and so on, and transmit this information to the brain or spinal cord. The brain or spinal cord then sends back messages through special motor cells, instructing the body how to respond—by pulling one's hand away from a flame, for example.

The sensation of touch is easily tested with a simple hat pin, a wisp of cotton, and so on, as will be described. Interpreting these tests, however, is not a cut-and-dried matter. There is a wide variation of normal response to sensory inputs from one person to another. The touch of a magician, a surgeon, a pianist, a safecracker, a pickpocket, or a card shark is likely to be more acute than that of the average person, yet all are within the normal range of response. Bear in mind, too, that some parts of your body are more discriminating than others. For instance, the fingertips are more sensitive than the back, the lips more than the top of the head, and the elbows more than the shin. Thus you would be mistaken to conclude that your sensory system was impaired simply because your lips detected a lighter touch than your shin. If, on the other hand, you discover that one foot is considerably more sensitive to touch than the other, this may be a significant finding. Many nervous-system disorders affect one side of the body more than the other; thus a marked difference in sensory response from side to side should be viewed with suspicion.

Testing Tactile Sensation

Superficial, or light, touch is very different from the firm pressure of, say, a handshake. Testing this sensation requires an assistant with a delicate touch; even light pressure exerted by a finger or hand in administering the test should be avoided.

1. Using a wisp of cotton or a soft, camel-hair brush, have your assistant lightly touch or brush various areas of your arms and legs, first on one side and then the corresponding points on the other side of the body.

2. With your eyes closed, report each time a light-touch sensation is felt. In rating your response, try to compare your sensitivity from side to side. A consistent pattern of missed responses on one side of the body is more significant than random misses on both sides.

Testing Superficial-Pain Sensation

Superficial-pain sensation is another distinct sensory input to the nervous system. Superficial pain is merely a light, fleeting irritation of the surface of the skin, not a deep or throbbing pain such as you would experience with a cut or a minor burn. A light pinprick is usually used to check superficial-pain sensation. You will need a large hat pin with a little knob at one end for this test, and an assistant.

1. With your eyes closed, ask your assistant to lightly touch various places on your arms and legs, sometimes with the point of the hat pin and sometimes with the blunt, knobby end.

2. Pay particular attention to examining hands and feet. Report each time you feel a touch, specifying whether it feels sharp or dull.

3. You should be correct most of the time. Your assistant should retest any areas where you give an incorrect report. Areas in which you consistently give an incorrect report or fail to perceive any sensation at all should be brought to the attention of your doctor.

Testing Stereognostic Sense

Testing another kind of sensory input to the nervous system, called stereognostic sense, checks your ability to "decode" sensory information. Stereognostic sense allows you to identify an object by touch alone, without looking at it. You can test this sense by providing your assistant with an assortment of small objects such as a penny, a quarter, a fifty-cent piece, a key, a marble, a safety pin, and a ring.

1. Ask your assistant to place these objects in your hand one at a time.

2. With your eyes closed, you should be able to report which object you are holding without looking at it. If you can do this, then you have normal stereognostic sense. You should also have normal two-point discrimination because these two functions really go together. Two-point discrimination is simply the ability to be aware that you are being touched at two nearby places at the same time. You can tell the difference, for example, if someone touches you with one finger or two.

The ability to detect hot and cold sensations and react appropriately is one of the nervous system's most important sensory inputs. Without it, our body could be irreparably damaged before the smell of singed flesh or the tingling numbness of frostbite alerted our brain to take action. It is no coincidence that one of the earliest words in every baby's vocabulary is "hot!"

Our skin registers different temperature sensations through special nerve endings, some of which respond to cold and falling temperatures, and others to heat and increasing warmth. The heaviest concentration of cold receptors lies in exposed areas such as the face, with emphasis on the tip of the nose, the eyelids, lips, and forehead. Parts of the chest, abdomen, and genitals are also highly sensitive to cold. That's why it's always easier to get your feet wet than the rest of your body when you go swimming. You are more sensitive to warmth, on the other hand, on the hairy parts of your head, around your kneecaps, and on your tongue.

Testing Temperature Sensation

Temperature sensation can be tested using two test tubes or two tiny glass bottles, such as single-serving whiskey bottles. (Don't use plastic bottles because they don't transmit heat well.)

1. Fill one tube with cold water and the other with hot water, about as hot as it comes out of the tap.

2. Have your assistant lightly touch these bottles to various parts of your body,
sometimes one bottle and sometimes the other.

3. You should be able to report with your eyes closed whether the hot or cold bottle is touching you. In some neurological disorders, a person may lose the sensation of cold altogether but still be able to sense warmth. In such cases, ice cubes placed on the skin will feel warm.

Testing Position Sense

Position sense is the ability to know where various parts of your body are without looking. This is possible because impulses from special nerve cells, called sensing or sensory cells, feed signals into the central nervous system that let you know almost instantly that you've raised your hand or moved your foot. You can check position sense in both your arms and legs in the following manner.

1. Arms: Close your eyes and touch the tip of your nose with your index finger, first with one hand and then with the other. Start with your arm extended straight out and bring it slowly in toward the nose. A near miss counts as passing, particularly if you can improve your performance with just a little practice.

2. Legs: While sitting in a chair with your eyes closed, touch the heel of one foot to the shin of the opposite leg and run it up and down a bit. If you can do this accurately with each foot, position sense in the legs is normal. As with the finger-

to-nose test, your performance may improve slightly with a little practice.

Testing Movement Sense

A final test that you can perform to check sensory functioning of the nervous system has to do with movement sense. To test this, you will again need your assistant.

1. Ask your assistant to passively move one of your fingers or toes while you have your eyes closed. Your assistant moves one of your fingers or toes up or down or to one side or the other just a little, being very careful not to touch one of the adjacent digits during the examination.

2. Each time a movement is made, you report the direction of the movement. You should be able to distinguish a movement of less than a quarter of an inch in any direction without too much trouble.

Motor Functioning

The nervous system controls motor functioning—that is, body movement—by signaling the muscles to relax or contract. It does this by sending impulses from the brain or spinal cord to the muscles through special nerve cells called motor cells. The fine fibers that trail out from each motor cell branch off at their endpoints to make contact with fine strands of muscle. The impulses sent through these motor fibers trigger the release of tiny amounts of a chemical that starts the muscle contracting. When the impulses cease coming, the mus-

cle relaxes. Motor function, then, or body movement, is initiated by these special motor nerves that direct muscle action.

Any abnormality of the motor system could, of course, be caused by a problem with the muscles themselves, and testing of this aspect of motor activity is covered in Chapter 8, which deals with bones, muscles, and joints. A neurologist, however, will perform special tests to determine that the nervous system is doing its job in directing motor activity. Some of these tests you can perform yourself.

The most familiar of all neurological tests, the knee-jerk reflex, tests the nerves supplying the knee, or patellar, tendon. As noted earlier in this chapter, the knee-jerk test is actually a test of a nerve loop to the spinal cord. The knee-jerk reaction is called a simple reflex arc because the nerves that receive the tap from the little rubber hammer send the signal to the spinal cord; the signal is processed right there and the message directing the muscle to jerk is sent right back. The absence of the knee-jerk reflex is usually a sign of nerve damage, particularly if it is missing on one side only.

Reflex testing is usually performed using a small, rubber-headed hammer. In the United States, the head of this hammer is usually triangular in shape and either the wide or the pointed end is used, depending on the preference of the examiner. There is, however, wide variation in the shape of these hammers. In practice, almost any little weight on the end of a short arm will do. If you wish to purchase a reflex hammer, they are widely available at medical-supply stores and are relatively inexpensive. If you are careful and gentle, any small tack hammer will do. Do not use a large carpenter's hammer or other dangerous tool. With practice, some people can learn to use the side of their open hand as a kind of hammer.

Testing the Knee-Jerk Reflex

1. The knee-jerk test is best carried out with some help from an assistant. Sit on a table so that your legs swing freely from the knee joint, with your knees bared.

2. Locate your kneecap with your fingers. This is the roundish bone that sits right over the knee.

3. Next, locate a bony prominence an inch or so below the kneecap. This is the top end of the large bone in your lower leg. In the very front part of your leg you will feel a fairly stiff cord running in the short space between the bottom of the kneecap and the top of the leg bone. You should actually be able to put your thumb and index finger on either side of this cord. You are now holding the tendon you are about to test. Mark this point with an *x* using a felt-tip pen.

4. With the legs totally relaxed, ask your assistant to briskly tap each knee at the point you have marked. It is very important to relax or the test will not work properly. Remember, it is a *tap*, not a blow.

5. In most people, if the test is performed correctly, the lower leg will immediately give a little jerk.

The normal response in this test is extremely variable. Some people have very active knee jerks and others have such inactive knee jerks that it is difficult to elicit any response at all from the test. If you are having difficulty obtaining a knee-jerk reaction, it sometimes helps to hook your hands together, hold them up in front of your chest, and then try as hard as you can to pull them apart. While you are pulling as hard as you can, your assistant should repeat the test. This increase in general muscle tone often strengthens the knee-jerk response in those who normally have a relatively weak response. The most important observation, however, is not the strength of the response, but rather the equality of response on the two sides. Both sides should be about the same. A knee-jerk response that is substantially more active on one side than on the other is abnormal and a doctor's opinion should be sought.

Other tendon reflexes can be tested in much the same way. The Achilles tendon, for instance, responds well to a simple ankle-jerk reflex test. Like the knee jerk, this is best carried out with some help from an assistant.

Testing the Ankle-Jerk Reflex

1. Sit on the edge of a table so that your legs swing freely from the knee joint, with your feet and lower legs bared.

2. Locate the Achilles tendon with your fingers: First identify the heel bone on your foot. Just above the heel bone, on the very back of the foot running up toward the leg, is a very strong, fibrous cord. This is the Achilles tendon.

3. Mark an *x* with your felt-tip pen on the very back side of this tendon at about the level of the ankle.

4. With your feet totally relaxed, ask your assistant to place the fingers of one hand on the ball of the foot to be tested and press upward with gentle-to-moderate pressure. Your tendency will be to help your assistant by lifting your foot, but resist this. Try to relax and, if anything, press down ever so slightly rather than lifting your foot.

5. Now your assistant should strike your Achilles tendon with the reflex hammer. It takes a moderately hard tap to elicit a response; it can't be too gentle, but neither do you want to receive a damaging blow. The examiner should practice tapping his or her own Achilles tendon first to get the feel of the test.

6. In most people, if the test is performed correctly, the foot should jerk downward. Do the test several times until you get a consistent jerk with each foot. As with the knees, the ankle-jerk reflex should be equal on both feet.

Tendon reflexes are an important part of a neurological examination because they help the doctor decide whether an existing problem stems from the brain, the spinal cord, or the peripheral nerves. A lesion of a peripheral nerve or certain parts of the spinal cord, for instance, results in a diminished reflex response, whereas damage to other parts of the spinal cord or the brain results in an increased reflex response. As stressed previously, the equality of the reflexes on the two sides is the most important judgment to be made. Reflexes that are equal from side to side but apparently more brisk in the legs than in the arms are usually not a cause for concern. Generally, it is only when the reflexes become unequal on the two sides that a medical opinion should be sought immediately.

An overall assessment of motor functioning can be made simply by observing the subject walking and running. Simple as they may seem, standing, walking, and running are the end products of a symphony of coordination involving nerve impulses going to and from the brain and proper muscle functioning. Just to maintain balance, your feet must signal their position to the brain, which then instructs the feet to make any necessary adjustments to keep you from toppling over.

Observing Gait

1. Ask your assistant to watch while you walk, stop, turn suddenly, and walk in the other direction; then jog in place for a moment or two.

2. You should walk with an entirely normal gait, you should turn promptly without staggering, and you should jog easily on your toes, taking the weight of your body comfortably and alternately with each foot.

Actually, you are probably a far more sensitive observer of your own gait than any examiner could be, and you will be aware of even slight abnormalities if they occur.

The last phase of a neurological examination checks a person's general level of mental functioning. This is not an IQ test to find out how "smart" someone is; rather, it is a series of simple questions carefully designed to check memory of both the immediate and the distant past, awareness of the surrounding world, and ability to perform abstract reasoning as demonstrated by simple arithmetic problems.

Testing General Mental Functioning

This test is much less formal than the others; in fact, except for the arithmetic, the entire test can be administered in the course of a casual conversation. You need not ask the same questions as those that follow, as long as you check both short- and long-term memory and verify an awareness of major current events.

1. Checking short- and long-term memory: Some questions you might ask are: Who is the president of the United States? Who was president before him? What time of day is it? What day of the week is it? What is the date? Ask about important family dates or events.

2. Checking abstract reasoning: Abstract reasoning is tested with an oral arithmetic quiz. The subject is usually asked to do simple, single-digit additions. If these are answered successfully, the subject is then asked to count to thirty-three by threes.

3. The most difficult arithmetic test used by neurologists is the series-seven test. In this test the subject is asked to subtract seven from one hundred. He or she answers ninety-three and the examiner immediately asks the subject to subtract seven from that answer. When he or she answers eighty-six, the examiner again asks the subject to subtract seven from the remainder. This continues until the examiner has been able to assess the subject's speed and capability.

There is no question that many people find this test difficult, and it is designed to be just that. The test is also somewhat stressful. Thus while many people do not perform the test either very accurately or very swiftly, it gives the examiner some idea of how the subject performs under slightly stressful conditions.

And that essentially concludes a basic neurological examination. Bear in mind as you review your performance that, for all their seeming simplicity, neurological tests are very tricky to interpret. A response that might be considered abnormal for most people might be a normal variation in the case of a particular individual. It takes years of training and experience and keen observation to pin down the root of a neurological problem. So these tests are not intended to be diagnostic of any disease or ailment. If you can get them to work for you, they are good indications that all is well. And no one is in a better position to detect slight abnormalities than you are yourself. Any unusual findings you uncover as a result of the tests in this chapter can be brought to the attention of a specialist that much earlier, and that can be important.

Some Disorders of the Brain and Nervous System

Disorders of the nervous system can result from many causes: bacterial or viral infections, accident and injury, autoimmune reactions, or interruption of blood flow, and for some, as in the case of epilepsy, the causes are as mysterious today as they were thousands of years ago. Some of the following disorders are discussed in more detail elsewhere in this book, but because they are related to the brain and nervous system, we will mention them briefly here as well.

Epilepsy

In people with epilepsy there seems to be a general misfiring in the brain, but no one knows why. In a grand mal seizure, the affected person loses consciousness, becomes rigid, and then begins a convulsive jerking about, eyeballs rolling, possibly foaming at the mouth, and often expels urine and feces. It is a frightening episode to witness and when it happens in public you feel you want to do something, but all you can do is try to see that the person is not hurt while thrashing about. Call your emergency service. The seizure usually doesn't last very long, but the affected person will probably need to undergo rest and observation afterward.

Some children experience what are called petit mal seizures, which last only a few seconds. The child may suddenly stop whatever he or she is doing and stare blankly or blink rapidly and then resume whatever was going on after the episode is over.

Convulsive Seizures

Epilepsy-like seizures may occur as the result of disease, high fever, accident, and exposure to fumes or poisons. Such an occurrence in a sick person or anyone not known to be an epileptic is a medical emergency and the person should be transported to the hospital at once by an emergency medical service.

Neuritis and Neuralgia

Nerves can become inflamed for a wide variety of reasons from disease to accident or for unknown reasons. When it happens it is always painful. Unexplained pain, numbness, or tingling in any part of the body that does not resolve itself within a few days to a week should be investigated by a physician.

Infectious Diseases

Fever

A high fever in any disease can bring on convulsions, especially in children—a good reason to try to bring a fever down with acetaminophen and cool sponge baths when a child is ill. Some infectious diseases such as meningitis and encephalitis attack the nervous system directly.

Meningitis

Meningitis can be caused by a variety of microorganisms and is a medical emergency. Fever is high and there can be a fierce and unrelenting headache. Characteristically, the neck becomes stiff and painful and the affected person finds it difficult if not impossible to bend his or her head forward.

Encephalitis

Encephalitis, an inflammation of brain tissue, can be a by-product of diseases such as measles or whooping cough or the result of a microorganism spread by mosquitoes. High fever, over 103° F, pounding headache, drowsiness, unresponsiveness or stupor, stiff neck, and vomiting are all danger signs not to be ignored.

Noninfectious Central Nervous System Diseases

Progressive malfunctioning of the central nervous system can manifest itself in such diseases as Parkinson's, multiple sclerosis, and other diseases that cause the muscles and other body organs to malfunction. A discussion of these problems is beyond the scope of this book, but some of the early signs and symptoms of these diseases can be discovered with tests described in this chapter, which is why an abnormal finding in any of them should be called to the attention of your doctor.

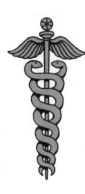

7

How to Test Your Urinary System

Urination is one of the most familiar body functions, but one that still isn't discussed much in polite company, despite liberated attitudes in other areas. Viewed with repugnance at best, the humble urinary system is taken for granted when it works and cursed when it doesn't. Like Rodney Dangerfield, it just don't get no respect! Moreover, because the end of the system shares space with the genitals, disorders of the two systems are sometimes related and sometimes confused. Women, especially, tend to confuse vaginal and urethral functions and symptoms, simply because of the physical proximity and obscured location.

Unhappily, disorders of the urinary system are often fretted over in private with a stoic fortitude that is quite unnecessary, because the urinary system signals its afflictions in a variety of ways that can be measured and tested with just a little attention and respect on our part.

Urination is one of the ways that waste is removed from our system. The parts of the body that are involved in this process are the kidneys, the bladder, and the tubes that connect them as well as the tube from the bladder to the outside of the body. Each kidney is connected to the bladder by a ureter. The tube to the outside world is called the urethra. This system is called the urinary tract, and it is the same in both men and women. The only difference is in the length of the urethra. The tube is shorter in women, and this is one reason women seem to suffer from bladder and kidney infections more often than men do. Men have their own problems, however, because their urethra is partially surrounded by the prostate gland. This is not part of the urinary system, but sometimes the prostate becomes enlarged and makes the passage of urine out of the bladder difficult. The prostate gland itself is discussed in Chapter 10, which deals with the reproductive system.

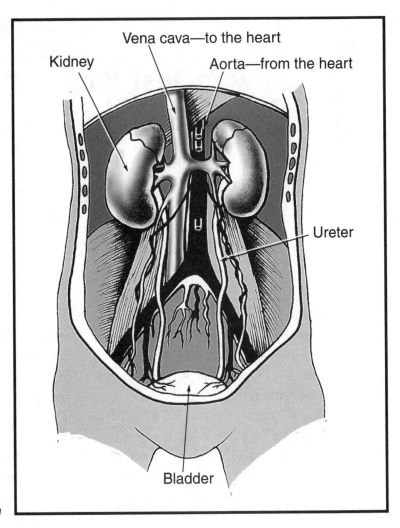

Organs of the Urinary System

Kidney Pain and Kidney Stones

The kidneys are located in the back of the body on either side of the spinal column. You can find the area where your kidneys are located by feeling for the edge of the lowest rib, just to the side of the spine. This point is known as the costophrenic angle. The prefix *costo* refers to the ribs; *phrenic* refers to the diaphragm. The costophrenic angle, then, is the corner formed by ribs and diaphragm. Some kidney diseases will cause pain in this area.

Testing for Kidney Pain

1. Make a fist and reach back and give yourself a few raps in the costophrenic angle. Just a good sharp rap will do; don't try deliberately to make it hurt.

2. If this blow causes pain, you may have kidney disease and you should see your doctor. And if this little test is positive, you probably experience pain in that area when you jump up and down or when you are bounced hard in your car as it hits a pothole or goes over railroad tracks. You need not have pain on both sides. Sometimes only one kidney is involved, and only that one hurts.

Cuts and bruises of the kidney resulting from automobile or other accidents or from athletic injuries may also cause pain. Many serious kidney disorders are painless, however, so the absence of costophrenic-angle pain does not mean that you are necessarily free of kidney disease. But if you do have pain in the costophrenic angle, this suggests a kidney disorder and you should have it looked into at once by your doctor. One caution: The back is heavy with muscles at this point, so don't confuse a muscle ache with the sharper pain originating in the kidneys.

Two of the things most likely to cause kidney pain are kidney infections and kidney stones. Many kidney stones are diagnosed on the basis of the clinical condition of the patient—that is, how you feel and how you describe your symptoms to the doctor. In most instances, small stones pass through the ureter into the bladder and out the urethra. The pain occurs as the stone passes down the ureter, and it is usually described as intense and agonizing. It can feel like an acute cramp that begins in the side or back and moves toward the genital region and inner thigh. The pain may last for several minutes or several hours. Women who have experienced both childbirth and kidney stones report that the pain of a kidney stone far exceeds the pain of childbirth. Other studies of relative pain intensity also give kidney stones a high rating.

Kidney stones are a perplexing topic, and many times doctors will not be able to determine exactly why an individual forms kidney stones. They just seem to happen. These stones form in the part of the kidney where the urine collects before running down the ureter. They are made of chemicals that, for some reason, do not stay in solution in the urine but precipitate out as crystals in the same way that sugar crystals sometimes form on the bottom of a maple-syrup can.

Once the kidney stone gets out of the ureter and into the bladder, the pain usually stops quite suddenly. The stone, however, may remain in the bladder anywhere from a few minutes to a few days. While the stone is in your bladder, you almost constantly have the urge to urinate and you find yourself going to the bathroom frequently and passing very small amounts of urine. This urge to go to the bathroom is also associated with infections. But if it occurs after a bout of superintense pain in the back, it is likely that it is a kidney stone.

Besides basing a diagnosis on clinical symptoms, doctors do further tests to confirm the condition. Most, though not all, patients with kidney stones have small amounts of blood in the urine. This is caused by the scraping the stone does to the inside of the ureter. The amount of blood in the urine is very small and not enough to make the urine look red or even pink. But these small amounts of blood are an important clue and can be tested for by microscopic examination or with a urine-reagent strip. Urine-reagent strips, available in drugstores without a prescription, are dipped in a urine sample and the color reaction is checked against a chart that comes with the kit.

X-rays are the best way to produce a positive diagnosis for kidney stones and will usually be recommended by the doctor when this problem is suspected. A plain x-ray of the abdomen will sometimes show a calcified kidney stone, but x-rays using opaque dyes that are injected into a patient's veins are the best way to find the stones. This x-ray is called an intravenous pyelogram (IVP) and is performed in a hospital setting.

Looking for Passed Kidney Stones

If you suspect you are passing kidney stones with your urine, it is a good idea to try to catch them.

1. Pass all of your urine into a container and then filter it through an old sheet or some other kind of cloth that will let water pass through easily. Cheesecloth is too coarse. Some stones are so small that they will go through the mesh of the cheesecloth.

2. Hopefully, you will find the stone. Sometimes it is no larger than the head of a common pin, and it is rarely as large as the knob on the end of a hat pin. If you find the stone, be sure to save it and take it to your doctor. Laboratory analysis of the stone will help determine the best way to prevent recurrence of this very painful problem.

Testing for Sugar, Blood, and Other Substances in the Urine

A number of substances may appear in the urine that are indications of problems in the urinary tract or elsewhere in the body. Dip-and-read tests (urine-reagent strips) have been developed to check urine for these various substances. These reagent strips are available in drugstores without a prescription. Instructions that come with the kits must be followed carefully and precisely, however, for them to yield accurate results. Not all brands of sticks perform all possible tests, so be sure that anything you buy includes the tests you want.

Sugar

Some doctors will check a urine sample for sugar as a screening procedure during a general physical exam. But if diabetes is suspected or if the doctor wants to check the sugar level in your blood, blood tests are more accurate. If you want to check your urine for sugar, you can use a reagent strip purchased in the drugstore.

Ketones

Diabetics who are in very poor control or who have not yet been diagnosed as diabetic will often show some ketones in their urine along with the sugar. Ketones are chemical substances that result from the breakdown of fat. This is not fat that you eat, but fat that the body has stored and is then using up. So the presence of ketones in the urine indicates that stored fat is being used by the body.

Anyone who is in a starvation state and is therefore mobilizing stored fat will show ketones in the urine. When very small amounts of fat are mobilized, the body is able to handle the ketones. When larger amounts of fat are being used, however, the body's ability to handle ketones is exceeded and they appear in the urine.

Ketones in the urine do not necessarily indicate disease. People on rather restricted weight-reduction diets often have ketones in the urine. One of the popular weight-reduction diets asks the dieter to measure urine ketones and suggests that only a positive result is proof of strict adherence to the diet. Anyone, in fact, who is on a diet that is restrictive enough to cause a substantial amount of fat mobilization will have some measurable amount of ketones in the urine. If you are on this restrictive a diet, you should be monitored by a physician.

pH

The pH is simply a measure of urine acidity. (You also measure pH when you test soil from your lawn or garden.) Seven is neutral; higher numbers are alkaline and lower numbers are acid. The pH of pure water is 7, and the fluids in body tissues stay close to a neutral pH 7. Gastric juice in the stomach, on the other hand, has a very acid pH of about 2. Normally, the body produces mildly acidic urine and a reaction of around 6 is not unusual. Certain diets and metabolic conditions may lead to the production of alkaline urine. Therefore, the pH measurement in any random sample of urine has little meaning. But if the pH is above 7, in the alkaline range, every time the test is conducted, this may be cause for concern.

Patients with chronic urinary tract infections often have persistently alkaline urine. The bacteria in the urine cause this to happen. And because bacteria thrive in a slightly alkaline urine, patients with chronic urinary tract infections are often advised to drink liquids such as cranberry juice that produce an acid reaction in the urine.

Protein (Albumin)

The presence of protein, also called albumin, in the urine may be a sign of serious kidney disease. A small amount of protein in the urine is normal in some people, but large quantities usually indicate kidney disease. People who spend nearly all of their working day on their feet, not moving around too much, sometimes have small amounts of protein in the urine. This is a normal phenomenon and is called orthostatic albuminuria. When the phenomenon was first described, streetcar conductors were often used as an example of the type of occupation that might give rise to orthostatic albuminuria. But now that example has to be replaced by a more contemporary figure. Perhaps someone who spends the day behind a supermarket checkout counter would be an appropriate choice.

Large amounts of protein in the urine may point to trouble, however. Children with a kidney condition called nephrosis often have large quantities of protein in their urine. Similarly, adults with various kinds of kidney disorders may have a significant quantity of protein present in the urine.

Blood in the Urine

Normally, blood is not present in urine. If blood does appear in the urine, it can come from the kidneys, the bladder, or any of the tubes connecting the various parts of the system. Passage of a kidney stone is usually associated with very small amounts of blood that come from the stones scraping against the walls of the ureter. The amount of blood is so small, however, that it can only be detected with urine-reagent strip tests or by microscopic examination.

Blood may also appear after a traumatic event. A hard blow in the area of the kidneys may injure them. This can occur with a football injury, in a fight, in an automobile accident, or in a serious fall. Microscopic amounts of blood may appear after minor traumas, such as a blow received in a football game, and will usually disappear within a few hours. Large amounts of blood indicate serious trouble, though, and a physician's advice should be sought promptly.

Disorders of the bladder will often make themselves known with bloody urine. And various kinds of tumors, infections, and erosions will produce varying amounts of blood in the urine. So bloody urine should never be ignored.

Not all red urine, however, is bloody urine. The urine can be colored red by many pigments. Sometimes food coloring will be excreted in the urine and will color the urine red without any blood being present. Beets, for example, will color some people's urine red when eaten in sufficient quantities. When women pass a urine specimen while they are having their menstrual period, it is often contaminated with blood, but this is not blood from the urinary tract.

The Odor and Color of Urine

The odor of urine may change markedly but it rarely has any medical significance. If there is an unusual odor about your urine, chances are it is related to some food you have eaten. The most striking example is asparagus. For many people, asparagus gives the urine a characteristically foul odor, while others may eat asparagus and have no noticeable change in their urine. Other substances also change the smell of urine, but to a lesser extent. In any event, none of these odors are anything to worry about, because except for a few rare diseases the smell of urine is not related to any particular illness.

Unusual colors in the urine, on the other hand, may be more important. As we noted in the previous section, a red color—if it is blood and not food coloring—is cause for serious concern and must be evaluated professionally at once. Very dark yellow or orange urine may indicate that one of the bile pigments is present in the urine. This happens in conditions such as hepatitis, which causes jaundice. Two tests are usually included in multiple urine-reagent strip tests—a test for bilirubin and one for urobilinogen—that show if substantial amounts of bile products are present.

Very concentrated urine may also be fairly dark in color without indicating any disease. Urine frequently becomes concentrated in hot weather, for example, if your fluid intake is limited. Some drugs can cause urine to turn blue or other unusual colors, which can be frightening if you have not been forewarned. If a doctor has prescribed the drug, you will probably be warned about what to expect. If it happens after you take a nonprescription drug, read the directions on the package or consult the pharmacist.

In a few rare diseases the urine is dark brown when passed, or it turns to a dark color when standing exposed to light. If you become concerned about the color of your urine, consult a doctor.

Bacteria in Urine

Of all the disorders that afflict the urinary system, infections are the most common. Urinary tract infections should not be ignored. Left untreated, they can eventually lead to long-term compromise of the kidney function.

A urinary tract infection occurs whenever bacteria find their way into the bladder. Urine normally contains no bacteria at all. Stool from the bowel, on the other hand, is loaded with bacteria, and it is not surprising that most urinary tract infections involve bacteria that come from the stools. Women get many more urinary tract infections than men because the urethra is much shorter and much more accessible to contamination by bacteria from the stool. Sex play involving both the anal and urethral openings, as well as soiled underwear, are common culprits in contamination of the urethra, so scrupulous cleanliness in these areas is important. Women should always wipe themselves from the front to the back after they have moved their bowels, because it is very easy to cause a urinary tract infection simply by wiping dirty toilet paper over the urethral opening. Wet wipes are useful when cleaning is difficult for some reason.

Several methods are available for the detection of urinary tract infections. Whenever you have the urge to pass urine frequently but only produce a small amount, you should suspect you may have a urinary tract infection. Pain or burning when you pass urine is a sign of infection. Although it is not terribly common, "silent" urinary tract infections can also occur. They are "silent" because the patient has no symptoms and does not suspect anything is wrong. This is one of the reasons that a routine checkup usually includes an examination of the urine.

The best test for a urinary tract infection is a urine culture. This must be performed in a laboratory equipped to grow bacteria. In this test, a small amount of urine is passed into a sterilized container after carefully cleansing the genitalia. Some of this urine is spread onto a culture plate and then incubated. If organisms grow, it is possible to identify them.

There are also dip-and-read tests that you can use at home to detect the presence of bacteria in the urine. It is best to do this test on a first-morning sample of urine. This will be relatively concentrated because you will not have taken in any fluid for a few hours and the bacteria will have had a chance to grow in your bladder for most of the night. You want a clean urine specimen for this test.

Taking a Clean Urine Sample

To obtain a clean urine sample, you should have a sterilized, widemouthed bottle ready. It is easy to sterilize the bottle. Just put it in a pot of boiling water for about five minutes. Boil the lid also if you plan to cover and save the sample to bring to your doctor.

1. Clean the area around the urethral opening well with warm water and soap. This is particularly important because you do not want to contaminate the urine specimen. Rinse thoroughly so that no soap lingers behind.

2. Have the bottle ready, but pass a bit of urine into the toilet first before collecting the specimen in the bottle. This is a further step to help avoid contaminating the urine. You now have a clean, first-morning sample of urine.

If enough bacteria are present, the test will be positive. This test can come up negative, however, even in the presence of a urinary tract infection if there are relatively few bacteria in the sample you choose to test. That's why in clinics and hospitals where laboratory facilities are available, a urine culture is the preferred method for testing for urinary tract infections.

Never let a urinary tract infection get a head start. Don't count on its "going away" because you drink a lot of liquids or because you use a patent diuretic medicine or folk remedy. Infections creep insidiously from one part of the system to another, and you want to avoid kidney involvement at all costs. Untreated kidney infections lasting even a week or less may cause serious permanent damage. So at the first sign of urinary tract problems, consult a doctor.

The Prostate Gland

The prostate gland contributes important nutrients to seminal fluid, the sperm-containing ejaculate produced by men during sexual intercourse. The design of the prostate, however, is generally counted as one of nature's engineering nightmares, for it is located at the base of the bladder and surrounds the urethra like a doughnut, where it can cause a variety of problems in a man's plumbing. When the gland enlarges, as it frequently does—especially in men over forty—it can effectively slow and eventually all but shut off the flow of urine from the bladder. If left untreated, severe discomfort and eventual damage to the bladder and kidneys can result.

It has been estimated that 50 percent of all men over the age of fifty are likely to develop some form of prostate trouble, and the risk accelerates with advancing age. Prostate disorders fall into three categories: benign prostatic hypertrophy (BPH), prostatitis, and prostate cancer.

Benign Prostatic Hypertrophy (BPH)

Whenever you encounter the prefix *hyper-* it means something is over or above. The suffix *-trophy* refers to growth. So hypertrophy of the prostate is simply growth or swelling of this gland. If it is benign, it is noncancerous.

The main symptoms of BPH all have to do with passing urine. These include difficulty starting the urine stream, a weak stream, interruption of the flow, and awakening frequently at night with the urge to pass urine, only to find there is little to pass. (This may occur more than twice a night, barring those occasions when you have had copious amounts of liquids to drink before bedtime.)

What is happening is that the enlarged prostate is pressing on the urethra it surrounds, preventing complete emptying of the bladder, or even preventing the passage of any urine at all. If ignored, this can lead to stagnation of urine in the bladder, backup of urine into the ureters and kidneys, infection, and serious impairment of the function of these vital organs.

There are several options for treatment of BPH, ranging from medication to a variety of surgical procedures, and more varieties of treatment seem to be emerging almost year by year. A urologist can fill you in on details and give you reading material to help you make an informed decision. You can also contact the American Foundation for Urologic Disease, 1120 North Charles Street, Suite 401, Baltimore, MD 21201, 800-242-2383.

Prostatitis

Infectious prostatitis is an inflammation of the prostate caused by a viral or bacterial infection. Because the prostate is pressed up against the rectum, pain from this condition may be felt as if it were coming from deep up in the rectal area. The pain often begins as something quite mild and gradually becomes worse. So if a deep persistent pain develops, it is important to see your doctor for treatment, usually with antibiotics. Prostatitis may also result in symptoms similar

to benign prostatic hypertrophy (described above), and in the case of acute prostatitis (of sudden onset) there may be chills and fever as well.

There is also a noninfectious prostatitis of unknown cause. It does not respond to antibiotics, so in this case the doctor will simply try to relieve the symptoms. Because symptoms of prostate cancer can resemble those of prostatitis, you should never assume that pain in this area will simply go away without verifying the condition with your doctor.

Prostate Cancer

Prostate cancer is second only to lung cancer as a leading cause of cancer death in men. In its early stages, when it is most curable, prostate cancer usually does not produce symptoms that would drive you to see a doctor. So it is imperative for men over forty to have an examination of the prostate conducted every year as part of a regular medical checkup. If your doctor doesn't offer to do this examination, ask for it.

The digital prostate exam, where the doctor inserts a well-lubricated, gloved finger into the rectum to palpate the prostate, is a subject of general embarrassment and locker-room jokes among men, but when all is said and done, it only takes a minute, causes little discomfort if you try to relax, and is all in a day's work for the doctor. What he or she is looking for are little lumps, nodules, or abnormal texture on the surface of the prostate, the same types of things a woman looks for in a manual breast examination that may warrant further investigation via biopsy—taking a sample of tissue from the suspect area for microscopic examination.

There is a blood test available to check for the presence of prostate cancer called prostate specific antigen (PSA) test, which looks for agents in the blood that generally appear when there are prostate problems. An elevated PSA finding, however, only indicates that further investigation or watching may be necessary. An elevated PSA can also be the result of prostatitis, and there can even be a normal PSA finding when cancer is actually present. So, currently, the digital rectal exam, or the digital exam combined with PSA testing, is still the best way to check for early prostate cancer.

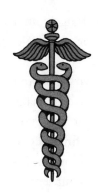

8

How to Test Your Bones, Muscles, and Joints

For most of us, the sum of our knowledge regarding the musculoskeletal system is contained in that familiar anatomical ditty that goes, "The head bone's connected to the neck bone, the neck bone's connected to the backbone . . ."

Actually, there's more to "them dry bones" than is suggested in this song, of course. For one thing, our bones are neither dry nor old—they are composed of living tissues that are continually dissolving and regenerating in an unending process that completely replaces every bone cell in an active person's body over a seven-year period. Furthermore, the bones and joints that make up our skeleton are only half of the great articular system that gives the human body its form and allows it to take action. The other half consists of the muscles, tendons, and ligaments that hold the skeleton together and allow us to make precise and subtle movements.

While bones perform a number of valuable functions, their role in body movement is largely passive—that is, they do not act independently but rather are acted on by the muscles that control them. Skeletal muscles are attached to bones at either end of their length and are left unattached in the middle. The attachments are generally made across a joint with one end of the muscle attached to a bone on one side of the joint and the other end of the muscle attached along a bone on the other side of the joint.

Any individual muscle is able to do only two things: contract to make itself shorter or relax. It does this in response to signals from the brain via the nerves that stream out from the spinal cord to the individual muscles. When a muscle contracts, one of the bones will move about the joint in the direction of the muscle pull. To get that bone back to its original position requires that the first muscle relax while another pulls from the opposite direction. Thus it takes a minimum of two muscles to move a bone about a joint and bring it back again.

In practice, however, a great many muscles are involved in moving any part of the body in any direction. It is this interaction of many muscles pulling in slightly different directions that allows the body to make subtle movements.

Consider your index finger, for example, and think of each muscle as a bundle of fibers that you can command to shorten or to relax. Now perform the following exercises with your index finger.

Observing Complex Musculoskeletal Movements

1. Hold your index finger out straight.

2. Bend just the middle joint without bending the end joint. This is a bit difficult but you can do it with a little practice.

3. Now bend the first two joints to curl your finger. Then bend all three finger joints as you do when you make a fist.

4. Holding the finger straight again, move only the third joint, the one where the finger joins the hand. Move the finger up and down and from side to side.

5. Flex just the middle joint and keeping the finger bent, notice that you can still move your finger from side to side.

6. Finally, bend and unbend the finger joints and move your finger in a circle at the same time. This is the kind of finger dexterity you need for buttoning a coat, playing a musical instrument, or

assembling the parts of anything from a model airplane to a computer.

Considering that at least two opposing bundles of muscle fibers are needed to make each movement, and considering that you have been moving only a single finger, you can get some idea of the tremendous number of muscles needed to give your entire body a full range of movement.

While many of the muscles that provide body movement are located along the bones they control, others extend a rather long distance away. For instance, the small muscles that allow you to make finely adjusted finger movements are located along the finger bones. But the big muscles that give strength to your grip originate up in the forearm. You can sense this by making a fist and feeling the action of the various muscles in your forearm, in the heel of your hand, and in the sides of your hand as you clench and unclench your fist.

Muscles are attached to bones by stiff cords of fibrous tissue called tendons. Where the tendons pass over a joint, they are enclosed in a tube called a tendon sheath. The inside of this sheath is very smooth and contains a small amount of slippery fluid that allows the tendon to glide smoothly over the joint. The joint itself is enclosed in a fibrous capsule that secretes a lubricating fluid that minimizes friction between the two bony surfaces that constitute the joint. And finally, the bones themselves are connected to one another at the joints by ligaments. These dense, fibrous bands maintain the bones in their proper relationship to one another and give the joint strength and resistance to sideward movement. Without ligaments, joints would fall apart whenever the muscles began to pull.

To review, then, the musculoskeletal system consists of the following five major components, and, as you will see, there are a number of tests you can do yourself to check on their functioning:

1. The bones that give the body its general shape and structure;

2. The joints between the bones that allow the body to be mobile and flexible;

3. The muscles that, with the help of the nervous system, provide all body movements;

4. The tendons that attach muscles to bones; and

5. The ligaments that hold adjacent bones together and keep the joints from separating.

The Bones

The bones of the body are hardly the inert girders that many people believe them to be. A typical long bone with the familiar, knobby ends consists of hard, compact bone on the outer surface, but spongy bone within and at either end. Bone marrow fills the hollow spaces in the spongy bone tissue and the narrow cavity that runs down the center of the bone shaft.

Bone tissue is composed of both organic and inorganic substances. The organic elements give bones flexibility and elasticity, while the inorganic constituents give the bones hardness and rigidity. The bones of young children have a greater proportion of organic material than those of adults and therefore are less brittle and more resistant to breaking.

If you listen to television commercials at all, you know that calcium is essential for bone strength. Both vitamin D and calcium intake are essential for depositing calcium into the bones. Fortunately for people in developed countries, milk (whether whole, low-fat, or skim) is an excellent source of calcium and most milks are fortified with vitamin D. If you don't or can't drink milk, you should consider a calcium supplement in your diet and vitamin D in the form of a multivitamin. Calcium depletion can result in osteoporosis, especially among menopausal women, and a regimen for preventing this should be discussed with your doctor during a regular physical and then followed rigorously. A drug has recently been approved by the Food and Drug Administration (FDA) that seems to remineralize the bones, but there is limited clinical experience with it at this writing, so continuing calcium and vitamin D intake is still advised, though you might want to discuss the new drug with your doctor as it may apply to you.

Growth and elongation of the long bones in children occur at an area called the epiphyseal plate. This is simply a soft growth area at either end of the long bones where the shaft, or center section, flares out to form the joint end. When this soft growth area is replaced by bone, near the end of adolescence, further growth ceases.

Most people's legs are very nearly equal in length. This is important because a difference of more than one-half inch can affect both your gait and your posture. When this happens, you must compensate for the short leg by placing abnormal demands on certain muscle groups in your body. In some people this can lead to chronic backaches and related problems.

A difference in leg lengths could be congenital, or it could be the result of abnormal bone growth following a fracture during the growth years. Or one leg may *appear* to be shorter than the other as a result of a muscle abnormality. In any case, a marked difference in leg lengths should be brought to the attention of your doctor.

Testing for Equal Leg Length

The best way to test for equal leg length is to look for pelvic tilt. You can do this by looking at yourself in a full-length mirror. The test is best performed while naked.

1. Stand up straight, facing the mirror, and place the thumb of each hand on the top of your pelvic (hip) bone. The top of your pelvic bone is on the side of your body a little below the rib cage. Your belt, when you wear one, usually hangs on it.

2. Check to make sure you are not standing at an angle but are facing the mirror directly. You should be able to draw an imaginary horizontal line between your two thumbs. If this imaginary line tilts up at all on one side, it may indicate that one leg is shorter than the other.

3. To be sure you are making your observations correctly, keep one foot absolutely flat on the ground and raise your other foot up on the toes a bit. You will notice that the thumb resting on that hip rises and falls as you raise and lower your foot. After raising and lowering your foot on both sides and watching your thumb rise and fall, again reexamine the relationship of your thumbs on both sides of your body. They should be exactly the same distance from the floor. If there seems to be a difference but you are not sure, enlist the aid of someone to measure the distance from thumb to floor with a tape measure.

Bone Tumors

Tumors can arise in bone tissue as well as in other body organs. These abnormal growths may be either benign (noncancerous) or malignant (cancerous), and if malignant, they may have originated in the bone or spread there from some other cancerous site in the body. Although there is a rule of thumb that cancer in its early stages does not hurt, the opposite is usually true of bone cancers.

Primary bone tumors (tumors that originate in the bone and have not migrated from some other place in the body) are most likely to appear in the long bones of the arms and legs. A benign tumor usually presents itself as a slowly progressing lump or bone deformity. Typically, the affected person first notices a hard, immovable bony knob or mass beneath the skin that slowly increases in size. This kind of tumor commonly appears near the ends of the long bones—above and below the knees are common sites—and is generally not painful, though it does hurt if bumped or bruised. Although such tumors are not cancerous, they generally should be removed, and if you find such a lump or mass, you should consult an orthopedic surgeon.

In contrast to benign tumors, malignant bone tumors are usually painful. Primary bone cancers are most common between the ages of ten and thirty and are unusual over the age of forty. Cancers that have started elsewhere in the body, however, and have migrated or metastasized to the bones may occur at any age.

There is one type of bone cancer (actually a cancer of the cartilage rather than of the bone itself) that has its peak incidence in middle-aged and older people. While bone cancers are most likely to strike the long bones of the arms and legs, cartilage cancers are usually found in the flat bones of the ribs and pelvis.

Bone Fractures

Bone fractures, usually resulting from some kind of trauma or injury, are among the most common bone disorders. A fracture is simply a break in the continuity of the bone. This break can take many forms, ranging from a simple break to a segmental, or double, fracture or even an open fracture that protrudes through the skin.

The exact location and severity of a fracture is generally confirmed by x-rays; in fact, some hairline fractures are virtually impossible to diagnose with certainty without x-rays. There are, however, some characteristic signs and symptoms you can look for when you suspect a bone fracture.

Diagnosing a Fractured Limb

The most obvious symptoms of a fractured limb are pain and an inability to use the injured part. Immediately following the injury there may be some numbness, but this will gradually disappear and the pain will become more intense. Movement of the fractured limb usually causes the pain to increase dramatically. Pain generally increases in severity until the affected extremity has been immobilized by a cast or splint.

In addition, the following observations may help confirm your suspicions:

- Tenderness at the fracture site
- Swelling at the fracture site
- Discoloration caused by bleeding into the tissue
- Muscle spasm; a muscle in spasm feels hard and tense.
- A visible deformity in a limb such as angulation—that is, a bend at an unnatural angle; if you are uncertain whether such a deformity is present, compare the injured limb with the limb on the opposite side.
- False motion or motion not at a joint
- Audible grinding of bony fragments during motion

Caution: Do not try to induce false motion or audible grinding. These symptoms should only be observed incidentally while the affected limb is being examined or while the injured person is being moved. Testing for motion of the two bony fragments can cause further injury to blood vessels or nerves. Do not try to set a fractured limb yourself. Managing this kind of injury demands more training than you are likely to get from a first-aid manual.

Diagnosing a Simple Rib Fracture

Thus far we have assumed that the fracture involves either an arm or a leg. Other bones, of course, can also be fractured. Rib fractures, for instance, are fairly common and sometimes difficult to diagnose. A major crushing injury to the chest is obviously a medical emergency, and you would have no difficulty in recognizing it as such. Lesser chest injuries, however, involving a simple, nondisplaced fracture of a single rib are usually much less apparent. Two tests are useful in diagnosing this kind of rib fracture.

1. First, simply observe the patient's breathing. A simple rib fracture often inhibits normal breathing. Someone with a fractured rib will tend to "splint" the injured side of the chest so that, when he or she breathes in, the injured side of the chest rises less than the normal, uninjured side.

2. A second test is to place one hand on the injured person's backbone and the other hand on the breastbone (sternum). Now press your hands together *gently*, as if attempting to press the breastbone toward the backbone. This would normally cause

the average person little discomfort. If the subject has a fractured rib, however, this maneuver will cause a sharp pain at the fracture site.

Diagnosing a Fractured Collarbone

Another common fracture involves the collarbone. The collarbone, or clavicle, is located just above the first rib, at the base of the neck. You have two collarbones, one on either side. This is a fairly common fracture site in children and teenagers and is usually the result of a fall or athletic injury. You can test for a fractured collarbone as follows:

1. The collarbone extends from the sternum in the center of the chest outward to either shoulder. A fracture of this long, slender bone is indicated by pain in the shoulder at the time of the injury that is made worse by subsequent movements of the upper arm.

2. Given these symptoms, hold the upper arm on the affected side tightly against the chest wall, supported upward just a bit. If this position relieves the patient's discomfort somewhat, a fractured collarbone is the likely cause of distress.

Other Fractures

Fractures of the back and neck pose special problems because they can cause extensive and permanent nerve damage to the spinal cord. The immediate handling of people with such injuries is very important. If you suspect someone has injured his or her back or neck, check for loss of movement or numbness in the limbs. If the person is unable to move an arm or leg or if a loss of sensation is apparent, do not attempt to move him or her by yourself. Call 911 for help. Serious further damage can occur in attempts to move someone with a back or neck injury.

Fractures of the skull or pelvis can be extremely serious. A severe blow or injury to either of these areas should be treated by a doctor at once. Transport by ambulance is advised.

Some pelvic breaks are obvious because of the pain and because the leg seems shortened with the foot rotated outward. The person can't stand and plainly needs help. But another kind of break, called an impacted fracture of the femur, happens in such a way that the person can get up and stand on it, giving a false sense that nothing serious has happened and that the pain will soon go away. If there has been a fall that results in serious pain that lasts for more than a day, it must be checked out at once and x-rayed for an impacted fracture.

So-called greenstick, or buckle, fractures are common in children, especially in the wrist. Children's bones are softer and more pliable than an adult's so that a bone may buckle and bend like a green twig on a tree and crack without breaking completely through. This kind of fracture heals quickly, but it is usually splinted or put in a cast by the doctor until it heals to prevent further injury to the same, weakened spot.

People sometimes come to an emergency room complaining of a painful hand, especially in the area above the little finger. They (most often men) admit to having hit someone or, in a fit of anger, punched a wall. It is, in fact, called a boxer's fracture. Some men, rather than investigating the pain, try to tough it out for weeks waiting for the pain to go away—which is not a good idea because a permanent injury or deformity can result from this kind of inattention.

In general, whenever there is pain, swelling, or inability to move after an injury, and certainly if there is any deformity in a body part, an examination by a doctor and an x-ray are called for. It is often very difficult if not impossible to tell the difference between a minor ankle sprain, for example, and an ankle that is broken without an x-ray being taken. Both can be sore and swollen. So if it's injured, painful, or swollen—or abnormal in any other way—don't guess that it will get better by itself without checking with a physician.

The Muscles and Tendons

Muscles, as explained earlier in the chapter, move bones. They are attached to bones by stiff cords of fibrous tissue called tendons. Any single muscle can do only two things— contract and relax—which it does in response to signals sent by the brain via the nerves that stream out from the spinal cord to the individual muscles. Because of this close association between the nervous system and the muscles it is often difficult to distinguish between disorders of the muscles and disorders of the nerves that serve them. A muscle may fail to work either because the nerve impulse to it is not being properly delivered, because of a nervous system disorder, or because the muscle itself is unable to respond to the nerve impulse. In such cases, even the experts must test carefully to determine where the fault lies.

Muscles and their tendons are also subject to a variety of common aches and pains that can be great or small and that may result from tension, unaccustomed or extraordinary use, fatigue, or injury. The causes of muscle and tendon hurts are usually obvious: overexertion without prior conditioning; a blow, a fall, a bad twist, or a pull; or a tension-filled day where the neck, shoulder, and back muscles seem to carry the weight of the world.

In most cases, muscle aches and pain of this type, even when they are rather severe, are straightforward and relatively easy to deal with. Rest, your favorite over-the-counter pain reliever, and reconditioning take care of most problems. Injuries to a tendon, on the other hand, or to the tissues where a tendon is attached to a bone can be a more serious matter. But let's look first at signs of muscle disease.

Muscle Disease

One of the earliest signs of a muscle disease is muscle weakness. Muscle weakness is a very gradual process that, for a long time, is most evident only to the person with the disease. Generally, one group of muscles is affected more severely than others, and many times such disorders involve one side of the body and not the other. In such cases you can test for muscle weakness by comparing muscle size and strength bilaterally—that is, from side to side.

Comparing Bilateral Muscle Size

With the exception of your arm muscles, which may be slightly more developed on one side, depending on whether you are right-handed or left-handed, the skeletal muscles of your arms and legs should be approximately equal on either side.

1. Measure the circumference of both muscles at their widest points. A fabric tape measure used for sewing works well for this purpose. Be sure you are measuring the muscle at the same point on both sides. It's a good idea to first measure up or down from some bony prominence before measuring the circumference of the muscle.

2. Compare your measurements; any difference greater than a quarter of an inch may be abnormal and should be reported to your doctor.

3. If a hurting calf muscle measures over a quarter of an inch more than the calf muscle in the other leg, deep-vein thrombophlebitis may be a suspected cause. (See Chapter 2 on blood, lymph, and the circulatory system.)

Comparing Bilateral Muscle Strength

Muscle disease affects muscle strength, too. Whether the muscle or the nerves that serve it are at fault, a poorly functioning muscle will lose tone and then strength over a period of time. You may be able to detect such a condition in your arms or legs by comparing the amount of resistance they offer when someone exerts force against them.

1. To help you spot muscle weakness in one leg, lie on the floor on your stomach with your knees bent and your legs forming a 90° angle.

2. Ask an assistant to grasp one ankle with both hands and try hard to bring the leg down to the floor while you use all your strength to resist.

3. Now do this with the other leg. Your partner should find it equally difficult—or equally easy—to bring either leg to the floor. That is, resistance in both legs should be about the same.

4. You can compare muscle strength in your arms in a similar fashion. Stand facing your partner with your elbows at your sides and both hands held out in front of you, palms up. Ask your partner to place his or her hands, palms down, on yours and press down hard, as if trying to force your arms down to your sides, while you do your best to

resist. Again, your partner should meet with approximately equal resistance from both arms.

5. If one limb is markedly weaker than the other, it should be brought to the attention of your doctor.

Testing for Myasthenia Gravis

Myasthenia gravis is a disorder of nerve and muscle function that in its early stages most commonly affects the muscles of the eyes and tongue and the swallowing muscles. Women are affected about twice as frequently as men and most often between the ages of twenty and thirty. An early sign of myasthenia gravis is a drooping of one or both eyelids; the following test assesses the strength of these muscles.

1. Sit comfortably in a chair with your head held in its normal position, facing straight ahead.

2. Without tilting your head upward, stare at the ceiling for a period of two to three minutes.

3. If all is well, you will be able to do this comfortably. Someone suffering from myasthenia gravis, however, will not be able to keep the eyelids open. Their eyelids will progressively droop until they cover most of the colored part of the

eye. After five to ten minutes' rest, strength will return to the eyelids, but on repeating the test the subject will again be unable to stare at the ceiling for a sustained period of time.

Muscle Spasm

Leg cramps, a "stitch" in the side, swimmer's cramps, a stiff neck, or the pain that can "lock" your back as you bend over to tie your shoelace are all examples of muscle spasm. Muscle spasm is usually an indication that a muscle or the nerves serving it are in a state of irritation for some reason: The muscle may be fatigued from overuse; the oxygen supply to the muscle may be insufficient to support the muscle's activity; the muscle or its tendon may be injured; or a nerve serving the muscle may be injured or irritated.

A disc problem in the vertebrae of the lower back can irritate a nerve, causing spasm in a thigh muscle or somewhere else in the back. Shin splints, a common affliction among joggers, is actually a spasm of the muscles of the front lower leg. Cramps in the calves of the legs or in the stomach, the severe kind that cause numerous drowning fatalities, are muscle spasms caused by muscle fatigue or inadequate blood circulation that disrupts metabolism in the muscle cells. In a sense, muscle spasm is a painful signal to stop using muscles that are suffering stress of some kind.

Leg cramps that happen in bed at night can often be relieved simply by changing position. Or getting out of bed and walking around may help.

Tendinitis

Tendons are the tough, fibrous cords that attach muscles to bones. When a particular muscle or muscle group is subjected to abnormal stress—such as hitting a tennis ball or wielding an ax—the shock administered to the muscle terminates abruptly in the tendon. Too many such shocks irritate the tendon and the site on the bone where the tendon is attached. This can cause a variety of tissue damages ranging from surface irritation at the site of attachment to actual tears in the tendon or the muscle tissue. In extreme cases, a tendon can tear away completely, pulling with it a portion of the bone or joint covering to which it is attached. Depending on the severity of the injury, treatment can involve simple surgery, immobilization in a cast, or just plain rest of the injured joint. Following recovery, the affected muscles will require rehabilitation in the form of special exercises to regain or, preferably, to exceed their former strength.

Joints and Ligaments

The joints of the body are the most complicated aspect of our musculoskeletal system simply because they incorporate so many different components in their functioning. Muscles, tendons, bones, and ligaments all come into play at the various joints to provide a wide range and variety of body movement.

As explained earlier, skeletal muscles are attached by fibrous tendons across joints so that when a muscle contracts, it can rotate a bone around the joint. This arrangement also

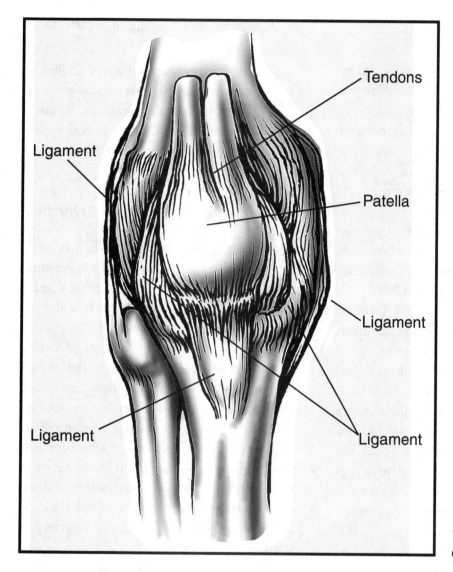

Tendons

Ligament

Patella

Ligament

Ligament

Ligament

Tendons and Ligaments
of the Knee

helps to hold one bone in its proper relationship to its neighbor. But the main holding force is the ligaments. Ligaments are tough bands of tissue that bind adjacent bones together at the joint, forming a fibrous capsule lined with lubricating membranes. In addition, joints are supplied with bursas; these are flat, lubricating sacs inserted between two adjacent structures—tendon and bone, tendon and ligament—to prevent rubbing of these parts. And some joints, including the knee and the vertebrae, are also equipped with discs of tough, cartilaginous tissue that act as cushions, or shock absorbers, between the bones meeting at that joint.

Normally, our joints can take a lot of wear and tear and still function smoothly. Unusual stress on a particular joint, however, or a breakdown in any of its contributing structures can unleash a wide array of miseries.

Arthritis

The suffix *itis*, you may recall, means inflammation, and *arthron* is the Greek word for joint. Arthritis, then, is an inflammation of a joint. This general heading encompasses a wide range of joint disorders stemming from injuries, infections, or just simple wear and tear on the contacting joint surfaces. Its effects can vary from mildly annoying to virtually incapacitating, depending on the nature and extent of the disease. Most cases of arthritis represent some form of either osteoarthritis or rheumatoid arthritis.

Osteoarthritis is the common arthritis of advancing age, generally making itself known after age fifty or later. Also called degenerative joint disease, this type of arthritis grows out of the accumulated effects of stress on a particular joint over a long period of time. The fingers and the weight-bearing joints such as the knees and hips are most commonly involved, and previous sports injuries to these joints make them particularly susceptible to osteoarthritis in later life.

Recognizing Osteoarthritis

A tentative diagnosis of osteoarthritis is indicated by some combination of the following symptoms and complaints:

- Aching pain in a weight-bearing joint (knee or hip) that is usually relieved by aspirin and a few minutes' rest

- Morning stiffness on arising that lasts a few minutes

- Occasional swelling of an affected knee

- Involvement of the fingers leading to deformities characterized by a knobby, twisted appearance. Knobs (Heberden's nodes) sometimes appear at the base of the finger joints.

Recognizing Rheumatoid Arthritis

In contrast to osteoarthritis, which is localized in one or more specific joints, rheumatoid arthritis, or RA, is a systemic disease that is apt to make its victims feel sick all over as well as sick at a joint.

Typically, the onset of rheumatoid arthritis is manifested by general fatigue, weakness, a loss of appetite, a slight fever, and vaguely defined joint and muscle complaints that escalate into full-fledged infirmity. This crippling disease generally affects much younger people—most often those between thirty and forty—than osteoarthritis does, and it strikes women almost three times as frequently as men. There is also a variety of RA that affects children.

The cause of rheumatoid arthritis is unknown and aspirin and other pain relievers are the usual treatment. Large doses of pain relievers must be used, however, and should be taken under the direction and observation of a physician.

Rheumatoid arthritis can be distinguished from osteoarthritis by the following characteristics:

- Swollen, inflamed joints in the hands, feet, wrists, knees, elbows, or ankles

- Reddened skin over the affected joints
- Morning stiffness lasting an hour or more
- Bilateral involvement—that is, the same joint is affected on both sides of the body
- Muscle weakness and atrophy in the affected area

Joint Injuries

Miscellaneous sports-related injuries to the joints are known variously as tennis elbow, surfer's knee, bowler's hip, thrower's shoulder, skier's heel, skater's ankle, and so on. Actually, while playing certain sports can produce characteristic injuries, you can also get tennis elbow from chopping wood, surfer's knee from scrubbing floors, and any of these other conditions simply by abusing a joint with prolonged and unaccustomed use.

Symptoms are pretty much the same for all of these injuries: pain, inflammation, and some degree of incapacitation of the affected joint. The pain alone will probably be enough to send you to the doctor, and it's just as well because injuries to structures supporting a joint can plague you in years to come if not managed correctly to begin with.

Most sports-related injuries represent some form of tendinitis, bursitis, torn ligaments, or some combination of these. You cannot diagnose the exact nature and extent of a joint injury yourself, but it helps to know what your doctor is talking about when he or she delivers the verdict. Here, then, are capsule descriptions of two of the most common joint injuries.

Bursitis

Bursitis is often a by-product of tendinitis, which we discussed earlier, and is often the result of overexertion by the weekend athlete. Bursas are small sacs of lubricating fluid found wherever friction occurs between adjacent structures, such as between muscle and bone, tendon and bone, or tendon and ligament. Their purpose is to prevent adjacent structures from rubbing on one another and interfering with the smooth operation of a joint.

Under normal conditions, the bursas function nicely. Repeated abnormal stresses at a joint, however, can irritate a bursa. When this happens, the bursa responds by increasing its production of fluid, causing the sac to swell. Because there is no extra space in the joint to accommodate this swelling, the swollen and inflamed bursa impinges on nearby structures. This condition is known as bursitis. It can be extremely painful and is most apt to occur in the shoulder or hip. Treatment consists chiefly of rest.

Torn Ligaments

Ligaments are dense, stiff bands of fibrous tissue that attach one bone to another at the joint and hold them together in their proper relationship. Without the necessary complement of ligaments to hold our joints in check, the bones would slide out of alignment. These should not be confused with the tendons that attach muscles to the bones *across* a joint.

Ligament tissue possesses a certain degree of elasticity that endows our joints with flexibility. Their elasticity is limited, however, and a severe blow or injury at a joint can tear some or all of the fibers that make up the ligament. This is what is called a torn or ruptured ligament or, simply, a sprain.

The most common sprains involve the ankle, as when you come down on the outside of your foot while running so that the foot turns inward under the ankle, or when a sudden force is applied to the outside of your knee, as might occur in a football tackle. Contrary to popular belief, a torn ligament is often *more* serious than a fracture, and if not managed correctly to begin with, it can result in chronic instability of the affected joint (trick knee, skater's ankle) plus further complications.

Because the symptoms of a pulled or torn tendon and a torn ligament are much the same, and because both are serious and potentially disabling, no assumptions should be made about an injured joint and no treatment should be undertaken without a careful examination by a physician.

Understanding Your Back

So far, our discussion of the bone, muscle, and joint disorders that can afflict the musculoskeletal system has excluded mention of the back, but not because our backs are immune to trouble. In fact, quite the opposite is true—the back is prone to such an array of miseries that it deserves a section all its own.

Your back is one of the most vulnerable regions of your musculoskeletal system. Not only does it have a large number of moving parts—there are twenty-six separate bones in the vertebral column alone—but the backbone depends on an intricate support structure comprising muscles, tendons, ligaments, and cartilage. Working together, they can bestow on us the flexibility of a gymnast. Let one element go awry, however, and you may feel its repercussions, literally, right down to your toes.

The central feature of the back is, of course, the vertebral column, or spine. This is a flexible column constructed of twenty-four separate vertebrae plus the sacrum and the coccyx—the last vestige of our ancestors' tails.

The vertebrae are divided into three groups. Starting from the neck down, the first seven are known as the cervical vertebrae. These are capable of an extraordinary range of movement that allows you to rotate your head from side to side and up and down. The next twelve are the thoracic, or chest, vertebrae, to which the ribs are attached. The brunt of the upper body's weight is borne by the last five, the lumbar vertebrae, and it is in this region that most back ailments are centered.

A typical vertebra consists of a round, flat bone and a pair of bony arches that meet to form a circular enclosure at one end. Three bony spurs project off this end of the vertebra, and you can feel the middle one, called the spinous process, as one of the bony bumps going down your back. When the individual vertebrae are stacked one on top of another, the circular enclosures form a canal down the vertebral column. This vertebral canal is the bony fortress that houses the spinal cord linking the brain with the rest of the body. The nerves of the spinal cord branch out to different parts of the body through openings in the vertebrae.

In between the vertebrae are those much maligned intervertebral discs, which are simply cartilage-walled capsules containing a resilient, jellylike substance. These discs act as shock absorbers, cushioning the vertebrae from direct impact with one another.

Each vertebra is connected to the one above and below by ligaments that serve the same purpose here as they do at other joints—that is, they maintain adjacent bones in their proper relationship.

The vertebral column is held erect with the support of three basic muscle groups that, together, act as guy wires with each exerting the precise amount of pull needed to hold the spinal column erect. Many major muscle groups in the back, abdomen, hips, and thighs work with the back muscles to give the torso its mobility and lifting and pulling power.

The entire spinal column, then, is actually a series of joints, complete with muscles, tendons, and ligaments just like any other joint in the body. While the large number

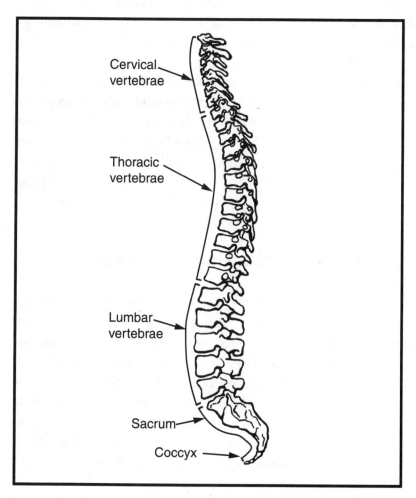

The Spinal Column

of joints allows us optimum flexibility, it also offers limitless possibilities for sprains, strains, aches, and related miseries of every kind. You should be able to diagnose some of these yourself or with the help of a friend.

Examining the Spine

The adult spinal column should be perfectly vertical, with a "lazy-S" curve when viewed from the side. This "lazy S" describes the four natural curves in the back: the cervical curve of the neck curves in along the neck to the shoulders; the thoracic curve reverses the cervical curve, curving outward to just under the shoulders; next, the lumbar curve is an inward curve again at the small of the back just above the buttocks; and the sacral curve completes the "lazy S" by curving outward at the bottom.

Checking Your Lumbar Lordosis

A potentially troublesome posture defect exists when the lumbar curve, or lordosis, becomes exaggerated. Excessive lumbar lordosis, also called swayback, may be caused by a genetic or organic defect in the spine or may simply indicate a weakening in one of the muscle groups that support the back. If not corrected, this condition can lead to backaches and even disc problems later on.

1. You should be able to spot excessive lumbar lordosis in yourself by critically observing your posture as viewed from the side using a full-length mirror or in someone else by simply inspecting his or her posture from one side.

2. The lumbar curve, as explained previously, is the inward curve of the spine in the small of the back just above the buttocks. Check to see that the abdomen does not jut out excessively in front, nor the pelvis in back.

3. If you or your subject stands with back against a wall, you should just barely be able to slip your hand into the space between your lower back and the wall. The greater the space between the lower back and the wall, the more pronounced is the lumbar curve.

4. If your posture shows an excessive lumbar curve, you should see your doctor for special exercises to correct this condition. Or many good books about the back are available that tell you how to strengthen back, buttocks, and abdominal muscles and reduce lordosis to a minimum.

Detecting Scoliosis

Whereas excessive lumbar lordosis is indicated by an exaggerated, inward curvature of the lumbar vertebrae, scoliosis is a side-to-side curvature of the spine. Normally, as mentioned earlier, the vertebrae should be stacked one on top of another in a perfectly vertical column. Any deviation of this column, either to the right or to the left, is abnormal, no matter how slight the sideward curvature may appear. This lateral curvature of the spine is called scoliosis and is most likely to develop in children between age ten and fifteen, with the incidence being much higher in girls and more common around age twelve or thirteen. No one knows exactly why this happens.

If detected early, scoliosis can be corrected with the help of appropriate exercises and/or a remedial brace. The condition "sets," however, at about age seventeen, and treatment after that is likely to be more drastic and the final results less satisfactory. For this reason, it is critically important that young people be examined regularly throughout their adolescent years for indications of scoliosis.

1. Have the subject stand up straight with his or her back bared to just below the waist. The little knobby protrusions running down the center of the back are the spinous processes of the individual vertebrae, as explained earlier. They should line up in a perfectly vertical column that does not deviate the least bit from side to side. Observe this column closely for signs of lateral curvature.

2. If you have any trouble locating the spinous processes, try this: Ask the subject to bend forward slightly from the waist; this will make the bony knobs more prominent. Then, using a black felt-tip pen, make a little dot on the skin directly over each spinous process (there are twenty-four). When this is completed, have the subject again stand straight. The little dots should form an absolutely straight line up the back.

3. A dropped shoulder is another indication of scoliosis. Observe the subject standing up with his or her back to you, again bared to just below the waist. Check to see that one shoulder does not drop lower than the other. They should be equal.

4. A variation of this test is to have the subject stand with his or her feet slightly apart and bend forward slowly at the waist, letting the arms hang down in front and keeping the knees straight. As the upper body drops downward, watch closely from behind to see if one side of the torso is higher than the other at any time. Normally, both sides should remain equal.

Checking the Cervical Spine

The cervical spine consists of the first seven vertebrae from the neck down. In addition to supporting the head, which is attached by ligaments to the top of the cervical spine, the cervical vertebrae permit the head to rotate 180° laterally and to look down at the ground and straight up. The nerves of the spinal cord that exit through openings in the cervical vertebrae serve the upper chest wall, the arms, and the hands. Pressure on these nerves, caused by disc disease or arthritis, for example, can cause symptoms that mimic angina pectoris ("heart pain")—discomfort in the chest that radiates down one or both arms. You can differentiate between heart pain and pain originating in the cervical spine with the following test:

1. Touch your chin to your chest. If this movement causes abnormal sensations in the upper chest, arms, or hands, and if tilting your head way back relieves the discomfort, you may have a problem with the cervical vertebrae.

2. Now touch your chin to each shoulder and then each ear to your shoulder. If any of these movements reproduces your symptoms, the upper spine rather than the heart is the likely offender.

Degenerative Disc Disease

One of the most troublesome of all back problems is degenerative disc disease, commonly referred to as "slipped disc." The spinal column, as you will recall, is made up of a series of small bones, the vertebrae, stacked one on top of the other. In between the vertebrae are circular capsules—the discs—consisting of a resilient, cartilaginous shell and a pulpy, gel-like center. If you can imagine a jelly bean inside a tiny tire casing, the consistency of the layers might be about right. The discs function as shock absorbers between the vertebrae, expanding and compressing in various directions as you twist, bend, jump, and strain.

Healthy discs can take a lot of abuse. But a degenerated disc is a calamity waiting to happen. Doctors are not always clear as to why a disc degenerates. Age is one factor—as we grow older, the discs become less resilient. But then, young people suffer from slipped discs, too. Poor muscle tone in one of the muscle groups that support the back certainly may be a contributing factor. Key muscles that aren't doing their jobs place abnormal strains on the spine and induce slight but potentially devastating changes in the relationship of the vertebrae, the discs, and their associated structures. And, of course, an accident or injury can damage a disc.

Whatever the underlying cause, the casing of a degenerated disc capsule eventually protrudes into the spinal canal or even ruptures, allowing some of the pulpy center to ooze out. When the oozing material causes pressure on a nerve or nerves of the spinal column, this creates pain, which sends your muscles into spasm and you to bed.

Fortunately, slipped discs are not nearly so common as simple muscle strain. Both of them can put you out of commission for considerable lengths of time and make you acutely miserable, but it is important to recognize a true slipped disc so that you do not further aggravate the condition with improper treatment. Exercises and treatments that may relieve pain caused by sore or injured muscles may cause severe nerve injury where a disc is involved.

Because discs do not show up on standard x-rays, actual verification of a slipped disc is obtained by magnetic resonance imaging (MRI). But generally, slipped discs are first diagnosed symptomatically. Following are some simple tests you can do that may indicate the presence of a slipped disc. If your back problem seems to conform to this picture, you should consult an orthopedist, neurologist, or primary-care physician without delay.

Testing for a Slipped Disc

Slipped discs most commonly occur in the lumbar region comprising the lower five vertebrae that support the bulk of the body's weight. A slipped disc here almost invariably irritates one or the other of the sciatic nerves, which run down the back of the legs. The following tests are designed to demonstrate, either directly or indirectly, this irritation of the sciatic nerve.

1. Lie down on the floor on your back and, keeping your legs straight, raise first one leg and then the other off the floor as high as you comfortably can. Normally, you should be able to raise each leg about 90°, so that the bottom of your foot is facing the ceiling. If, however, you have a slipped disc, you will be unable to raise one leg more than 45° or so from the floor without pain. If you encounter such pain, *do not* try to fight it and force your leg higher; this will only inflame the already irritated sciatic nerve.

2. Standing with your legs straight, bend over and try to touch your toes with the tips of your fingers. An average person can get within a few inches of the floor or at least to the knees, whereas the victim of a slipped disc will most likely fall far short of even reaching the knees because of a painful pulling in the back of one leg. If such a person were to try to touch his or her toes one leg at a time, he or she would perform much better on one side than the other.

A long-standing disc problem can result in varying degrees of neurological deterioration indicated by weakness, numbness, tingling, or decreased reflexes in the affected leg, possibly as far down as the foot. To check for this, refer to Chapter 6 on the nervous system. Four tests there may be helpful to you in determining whether one leg has been affected by chronic disc disease. They are: "Testing Tactile Sensation," "Testing Superficial-Pain Sensation" (you should be testing the feet and legs in both cases), "Testing the Knee-Jerk Reflex," and "Testing the Ankle-Jerk Reflex." The most important judgment to be made when carrying out these tests is equality of response—your reflexes should be equally strong in both legs, and both limbs should be equally sensitive to pinpricks and light-touch sensations.

A painful disc condition with sciatica can also, over a period of time, result in a loss of muscle tone in the affected leg. To check for this, you should compare bilateral muscle size and strength in the calves or thighs, whichever seems to be affected by your ailment, using the muscle tests described earlier in this chapter.

Not every slipped-disc sufferer will exhibit all the symptoms indicated by these tests. But persistent backaches accompanied by pain in one buttock and down the leg, plus a positive response to any of the tests described, should be enough to send you to a specialist.

Surgery for degenerative disc disease was much more common a few years ago than it is today. Most physicians nowadays prefer to first try a more conservative approach to the problem and resort to back surgery only after other therapies have failed. Physical therapy can provide relief, and many people are helped by chiropractors or by using other forms of alternative medicine. Plain old rest and care in exercise and lifting often works, too. As long as a part of the disc is not pressing on a nerve coming out of the spinal column, conservative treatments can be very effective.

A Checklist for Back Problems That Are About to Happen

Some back problems result from a single accident, but most develop slowly over the years as a result of deterioration of muscles that support the back (back, hip, and abdominal muscles) and as a result of misusing and abusing the back. If you answer yes to three or more of the following questions, chances are good that if you don't already have back problems you soon will.

- When you stand naturally with your heels and shoulders against a wall, can you slip your clenched fist between the wall and the small of your back just above the buttocks? (This is too much lordosis and indicates poor posture.)

- Do you regularly sleep on your stomach or spend long periods of time lying on your stomach?

- Do you pick up items from the floor (even small ones) by bending forward from the waist without bending your knees?

- Do you bend forward from the hips with your knees stiff when you lift packages from the trunk of a car?

- Does your job require long hours of standing or sitting without adequate back support?

- Do you spend long hours in a chair where your upper legs slant downward from your hips to your knees?

- Do you frequently have to lift heavy items from a shelf or platform that is higher than your waist?

- Do you frequently have to lift a heavy object and twist your body to place the object somewhere?

- Are you more than ten pounds overweight?

- Perform the minimum strength and flexibility tests at the end of this chapter. Did you fail any of them?

- Are your stomach muscles flabby and paunchy?

- Do you exercise less than twice a week?

- Do you engage in a sport (without prior back-muscle conditioning) that requires sudden and severe twisting of the torso (golf, tennis, football)?

Actually, even *one* yes answer represents an abuse of your back that can lead to back instability and consequent back ailments. If you have several yes answers you would do well to read one of the many "back" books available in most libraries. If you already have severe and chronic back problems or if your back is frequently subjected to abuse, you should discuss corrective measures with a professional.

Tests for Minimum Strength and Flexibility

The ultimate test of the musculoskeletal system is, of course, how well it serves you in your daily life. At the very least, your body should be strong enough to allow you to cope with normal demands likely to be put upon it. Unfortunately, even this modest goal is seldom realized. In fact, it has been estimated that more than half of all Americans—young and old—cannot meet even minimum standards of physical strength.

The following five tests were designed to determine the minimum physical strength and flexibility required for ordinary people in routine daily living. They provide a yardstick by which to assess the basic well-being of your musculoskeletal system. The tests are simple, and they are safe for healthy people of all ages. (If you are convalescing from an illness or if you suffer from back problems, you should not attempt these tests without first checking with your doctor.)

1. Lie down on the floor on your back with your hands on the floor, palms up, next to your neck. Keeping your legs straight, you should be able to raise them approximately ten inches off the floor and hold them there for ten seconds.

2. Lie down on the floor on your back with your knees bent and your feet secured under a couch or chair or held down by a partner. You should be able to roll up to a sitting position.

3. Lie down on your stomach with a pillow placed under the pelvic area and your feet held down securely. With your hands behind your neck, raise your head and chest off the floor and hold this position for ten seconds. Do not overarch your back doing this—it is enough if the torso just clears the floor.

4. Lie face down on the floor once again with a pillow under your pelvic area. You will need a partner to press down on your upper back to hold your chest to the floor. From this position you should be able to raise your legs off the floor, keeping them straight, and hold them there for ten seconds.

5. Finally, you should be able to bend over from the waist and, keeping your legs straight and feet together, touch your fingertips to the floor (or almost).

As simple as these tests may seem, it is amazing how many people cannot meet even these minimum standards of strength and flexibility. If you can't do any of these tests, you should seriously consider enrolling in a reputable fitness program. Getting into shape is easier than you think, and the benefits to your musculoskeletal system and other body systems may well give you that extra measure of vitality you need to work and play as hard as you wish.

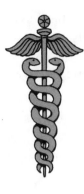

9

How to Identify Skin Blemishes and Ailments

The skin is the great envelope that wraps the body; it is our largest organ, constituting 15 percent of our body weight, and it is the most visible aspect of ourselves that we present to the outside world. So we pamper our skin, worry over it, and bemoan every spot that detracts from its loveliness. We worry so much about our skin, in fact, that severe, widespread blemishing, such as occurs in acne or psoriasis, can cause marked personality changes in its victims.

Trauma that destroys as little as 10 percent of the skin covering the body has serious medical consequences, and if something more than half the skin is damaged by burns or other injury, the chance of death, even with careful management, becomes substantial. Consider how many functions the skin performs:

- Skin is a protective shield and a waterproof overcoat for the body. It prevents noxious elements in the environment from getting at more delicate tissues underneath. Skin pigment protects us from the damaging effects of ultraviolet rays from the sun.

- Skin prevents loss of vital fluids and other substances from within the body.

- Skin is a thermal shield and helps in the regulation and maintenance of body temperature.

- Skin is an excretory organ, helping to rid the body of excess water and waste materials.

- Skin contains nerves that enable us to feel through touch and alert us to danger from invasion or changes in temperature.

- Skin is a factory that produces essential vitamin D.

We use our skin extensively in nonverbal communication of our emotions: We wrinkle the skin in different ways to express joy or sorrow, worry or anger; the skin blushes with embarrassment and blanches with shock or fear. Skin is an identification factor in its color and in the distinctive patterns it forms on the hands and feet; it tells our age and sometimes gives us a characteristic odor. Skin and hair are sexually attractive; skin touching is sexually stimulating, comforting, and reassuring. And the appearance of the skin can provide important information about the general state of one's health.

Rashes occur with many illnesses that affect the body systems—measles, chicken pox, and secondary syphilis are among these. Chronic itching may herald anything from nervousness to serious disease. Discoloration of the skin may point to disease—yellowing in jaundice and darkening in Addison's disease. Excessive and inappropriate sweating can result from simple nervousness, drugs, alcohol, or a hormonal imbalance. Sweating on only one side of the body may tell of nerve or brain damage, while hot, dry skin can tell of fever or sunstroke.

You may have noticed that one of the first things a doctor does in performing a general examination is to take your hands and gently look first at one side and then the other. He will rather caressingly run his hand over your arm and perhaps your back. This does two things—it calms you and establishes rapport through touching, and it provides a wealth of information about you and your general physical condition.

The Structure of the Skin

The skin is composed of three layers. The top layer, called the epidermis, is the part most often thought of as being typical skin. It has two main types of cells, keratinocytes and melanocytes. The keratinocytes produce a special material called keratin, which is a system of threadlike filaments imbedded in a nonstructured, gluey substance. This gives the skin toughness that enables it to withstand a good deal of pounding and scraping.

The other important cell type in the epidermis is the melanocyte. These cells produce pigment, called melanin, and, as you might expect, people with dark skins have a large number of active melanocytes, whereas people with fair skins have fewer or inactive cells of this type. Tanning after exposure to the sun is caused by increased amounts of melanin in the skin.

The middle layer of the skin is called the dermis. This is filled with a variety of structures that serve the skin and the rest of the body in a number of ways: connective tissue, which gives strength and resiliency to the skin; blood vessels, which nourish skin cells and carry waste materials to the skin to be disposed of; nerves, which detect touch and temperature change; oil glands; sweat glands; hair follicles; and tiny muscles.

The epidermis and the dermis lie atop a layer of fat, sometimes called the subcutaneous tissue (meaning "under the skin"), that acts as a cushion and shock absorber for the skin and separates it from the underlying muscle and bone. Skin can be as much as a quarter-inch thick over the soles of the feet or as thin as one-fiftieth of an inch over the eyelids and the eardrums. The subcutaneous fatty tissue adds thickness in most places around the body with the exception of such sites as the shins and the outer shells of the ears where you can feel bone and cartilage directly underneath the skin.

The outermost cells of the epidermis, called the *stratum corneum*, or horny layer, are actually dead cells that constantly dry and fall off. These cells are replaced by others that migrate to the surface from underneath in a process that goes on continually. New cells are produced at the bottom of the epidermis and slowly die, flatten out, and move to the surface of the skin. The full cycle takes a little less than a month, which means that you replace the outer layer of the skin about twelve times a year. This process is highly visible when you see the outer surface of the skin peel in large flakes after having been burned by the sun. Both hair and fingernails, incidentally, are made up of these dead epidermal cells that have undergone specialized changes.

Examining Your Skin and Tracking Skin Health

Dermatology is the medical specialty that deals with disorders of the skin. The dermatologist depends mostly on keen powers of observation and extensive training in recognizing several hundred kinds of skin disorders. So most tests for skin disease are simply very close observations of the nature of the lesion being dealt with. A detailed medical history and close questioning about a person's habits and environment are also essential ingredients that go into a dermatologist's diagnosis. Sometimes the dermatologist uses a magnifying glass to help see the exact structure of a lesion; he or she may arrange the examining lights to either create or elim-

inate shadows, and he or she may use a longwave ultraviolet light called a Wood's light that helps to detect fungal infections and some disorders of skin pigment.

The dermatologist also uses the laboratory, either sending skin scrapings out for analysis or making on-the-spot microscopic examinations. The dermatologist frequently resorts to skin biopsies for diagnosis of suspicious lesions. This is accomplished by applying a local anesthetic and then taking a circle of skin, including part of the lesion, with a little round cutting tool called a biopsy punch. This sample then is sent to a pathology laboratory for examination. A normal complement of blood tests is also used to diagnose some skin problems.

Because similar skin disorders may originate in the environment, in a person's system because of generalized disease, or even in a person's mind, the process of diagnosis will often challenge the imagination of a Sherlock Holmes and the wisdom of a Solomon. Another consideration for a doctor when diagnosing skin problems is the color of the patient's skin. Redness or shades of brown, for example, are markers in many skin conditions, and it is sometimes more difficult to see these colors superimposed on dark-colored skin. So if your skin is dark, you want to be sure that your dermatologist or primary-care physician has experience in examining patients with your skin tone.

Treatment may be as simple as changing an irritating laundry detergent or as complicated as managing a broadside of medications. Obviously, then, an untrained person cannot do the job of a dermatologist for him- or herself or for anyone else. But it is definitely useful and sometimes can be lifesaving to know your skin and to keep track of what it is doing. So part of your health-tracking procedure should include close, systematic observation of your skin, and records should be kept of your skin condition and the location and size of any blemishes.

Examining the Skin

To conduct a skin examination you will have to work with a partner because most skin areas are where you can't see them easily by yourself. Mirrors can help in a self-examination, but they don't allow the careful observations you need to make.

1. The examiner should follow an orderly routine so as not to miss anything. Begin with the hands: palms, backs, fingernails, and between the fingers. Then proceed from the top down: hair and scalp, face and neck, shoulders, trunk and arms, and so on. Be sure to check skin folds, armpits, the groin area, genitals, and other hidden places that provide exceptionally fine growing conditions for bacteria and fungi.

2. Make notes as you go. The examiner may talk into a tape recorder nearby or the subject may take notes as the examiner makes observations.

3. Try to notice and comment on everything, no matter how usual or insignificant it may seem. If you miss something such as "cool, dry palms," it may not seem unusual later if the palms change to moist and clammy.

4. Some things you should notice include: condition of the skin—rough, smooth, dry, oily, flaking; color—pale, flushed, uniform or nonuniform; marks, irregularities, and blemishes—bumps and lumps, moles, freckles, warts, age spots, sores, discolorations, bleeding or crusting, unexplained black-and-blue marks.

5. Note the size, color, and how long the subject has had the mark or sore. Measure blemishes with a small ruler, preferably one that is calibrated in millimeters. Use a hand magnifying glass to accurately describe the color, nature, and texture of blemishes.

6. Note complaints of chronic itching, evidence of scratch marks, or complaints of profuse sweating when there is no apparent reason for it.

Once you are aware of everything that is on your skin it is both interesting and informative to have all your observations explained. With notes and questions in hand, visit a dermatologist, have your skin examined professionally, and ask the doctor to explain your collection of lumps, bumps, and blemishes. At this time you can find out which are not worth worrying about and which you should keep an eye on. You may also find that some annoying blemishes can be gotten rid of rather easily.

It is not a waste of time and money to visit a doctor—even a specialist—when you are well. Specialists are so used to seeing patients only when they are in trouble that the doctor may wonder at your initiative, but once you explain your interest you are likely to be well received. Then, once you have an intelligent record, any disturbing changes that occur can be evaluated and treated quickly.

A change in a mole or a change in other blemishes is especially important and one of the American Cancer Society's cardinal signs of skin cancer. Melanoma, a particularly insidious and virulent form of skin cancer, often starts out from slightly raised skin lesions such as a mole or an age spot and, in the course of enlarging, changes from a medium to a dark brown to a bluish or dark gray color. But any skin blemish that changes in size, color, or texture should be evaluated professionally without delay.

Skin cancers are among the most common malignancies found in people, and the killer potential of melanoma can't be emphasized too strongly. Early diagnosis, which means early discovery, followed by removal of the malignancy is lifesaving. Once the malignancy begins to spread from its original site, death rates are high. Prospects for a cure are excellent, on the other hand, with early diagnosis and removal.

Danger Signs of Malignancy in a Pigmented (Colored) Blemish

- The appearance of varying colors should be viewed with suspicion. When colors such as red, white, or blue appear in any skin blemish, this must be investigated.

- If the border of a skin blemish becomes irregular, especially with noticeable notching at some point, this suggests trouble.

- When the surface of a blemish becomes irregular, bumpy, rough, or uneven, a developing melanoma may be suspected.

The diagnosis and treatment of skin disorders is an extremely complicated business. Many conditions have similar appearances and their causes are frequently difficult to ascertain and are often unknown. Therefore, any unusual eruptions should be called to the attention of a doctor. Because skin disorders can have causes other than skin dysfunction, other specialists besides a dermatologist are sometimes needed. Internists, allergists, the specialist in family medicine, and at times the help of a psychiatrist may be called on.

The blemishes and disorders described in this chapter are only a sampling of the woes a person's skin may fall heir to, but because they are the most common ones, you should have at least a passing acquaintance with them.

Moles

Moles usually begin as flat brown spots and then become slightly raised. They are simply clusters of melanocytes, the normal skin cells that produce pigment, and more than 95 percent of adults have them. In areas of normal white skin, melanocytes are widely scattered and produce only small amounts of pigment.

It is the clustering of these cells that produces the characteristic brown color of moles.

The reason that people are cautioned to watch moles for changes is that melanoma, the virulent skin cancer mentioned earlier, originates in melanocytes. Because melanocytes are all over the body, melanoma can originate anywhere, with or without a mole. But because moles are concentrations of melanocytes, the chances of a melanoma beginning in a mole are somewhat increased over other skin areas. A mole that does not show signs of changing, and that has been pronounced safe in the course of a regular examination, may be left alone unless you want it removed for cosmetic reasons.

Hemangiomas (Birthmarks)

Red patches on the skin may be present at birth or appear in the first year or so of a baby's life. "Stork bite" is a name given to little pink or salmon-colored patches that appear on the eyelids, the forehead, or the nape of the neck of newborns and fade away spontaneously in a few months or a year.

"Port-wine stain" can also be present at birth. It is a flat patch, colored red or purple-red, and may enlarge over the first few months before stabilizing. Except for the coloring, the skin is normal and rarely presents anything but a cosmetic problem. Occasionally, a port-wine stain indicates a blood-vessel abnormality, but your pediatrician will be aware of this and will advise you accordingly. Port-wine stains do not fade, but laser therapy may help in some cases. If they are in a noticeable place, cosmetic covering creams can help somewhat.

"Strawberry marks" may be present at birth, but they appear more frequently during the first month of life. They tend to be bright red and are raised. They may grow rapidly for a while, but then the majority of them disappear by themselves over a period of several years.

All these red markings are caused by a large collection of capillaries (tiny blood vessels) under the skin, so you can check rather easily to see if a red mark you are looking at is one of these.

Identifying Hemangiomas

1. Press down on the mark with a clear piece of glass you can see through. The bottom of an ordinary water glass will do.

2. Hold for a few seconds and observe the mark through the glass. If there is some blanching of the red mark where you press down, you are looking at an area of skin that is filled with tiny blood vessels—a hemangioma. Your doctor can tell you for sure what kind it is and what you may expect in terms of its staying or going away.

3. If the color does not blanch when you press down, it is probably a small bruise.

Liver Spots and Freckles

Liver spots, or lentigines, are similar to moles because increased numbers of melanocytes produce a characteristic brown-to-black color. But these cells don't cluster as they do in moles and so liver spots remain small and flat. They mostly inhabit the face and the backs of the hands and are probably related to exposure to the sun in the course of a lifetime. They are characteristic of aging but may appear early in life as well. Sun worshipers and people who work outdoors are likely to develop more liver spots earlier than people whose skin is protected from the sun most of the time.

The tendency to have freckles is inherited, and they seem to result more from highly active melanocytes than from clusters of them. After exposure to the sun, the melanocytes become large and very active, increasing the amount of pigment in the freckle spots.

Melasma

Melasma is a darkening of skin pigment in patches about the face and is strictly of temporary cosmetic concern because no other symptoms are involved and the patches of skin eventually return to their normal color. This frequently occurs in pregnant women or in those who are taking oral contraceptives, but the condition is also found on occasion in men, as well as in women who are not pregnant and not using oral contraceptives. It seems especially common among people with Latin origins.

A dermatologist can usually manage to lighten the darkened areas gradually so that when the condition disappears the skin will return to its normal color. Permanent skin bleaches should be avoided because they simply cause the opposite problem—white patches.

Vitiligo

Loss of skin pigment in patches that leave white areas of skin with sharply defined borders is called vitiligo. It is most commonly a genetic disorder that appears in families in an irregular inheritance pattern. For reasons that are presently unknown, the melanocytes in patches of the skin completely disappear. These patches may be tiny and barely noticeable or may involve large portions of the body.

A few other things can account for loss of skin color: injury, burns, certain fungal infections, and glandular diseases; but you are likely to know about an injury or infection, and a glandular disease will make itself known with other symptoms of illness.

Seborrheic Keratosis

This is a benign skin tumor that resembles a mole but becomes thicker and often looks like it has been stuck onto the skin. It may feel oily or rough and dry. These lesions seldom appear before age forty, and when large numbers of them occur, it may turn out to be a family trait. They are not harmful, but if they present a cosmetic problem or if they are a nuisance for some other reason, they can easily be removed by a doctor.

Skin Tags

Skin tags are little protrusions or polyps of normally colored skin. They resemble little nipples and may appear about the eyelids, the neck, and the trunk and in upper-body creases that occur with obesity. Skin tags are harmless and may be left alone, but if they are a bother they can be removed quite easily by a doctor.

Benign Cysts and Tumors

Lumps and swellings covered by normally colored skin may occur in any of the skin layers or in the fatty, subcutaneous tissue. These are known as dermatofibromas, wens, and lipomas. Any such lumps should be investigated by a doctor. If it is indeed one of the structures mentioned, it is no cause for concern and the doctor will probably leave it up to you whether you want it removed or not. However, if one is growing in a place where it might become a cosmetic problem in the future or interfere with wearing certain kinds of clothing, it is probably a good idea to have it removed sooner than later so that the resulting scar can be a small one.

Tattoos

People who have themselves tattooed should realize it is a lifetime proposition. Contrary to common belief, lasers and other modern methods for dealing with tattoos are not all that successful. These procedures may make a tattoo less obvious, but they may leave scarring or other skin blemishes. With tattooing, the skin has been damaged and cannot be returned to its original pristine loveliness at that spot again.

Diaper Rash

Called napkin rash by those who call diapers nappies, this is the first skin irritation that most of us experience, and it is caused by the irritating effects of urine and feces held against the skin by the diaper. The entire diaper area becomes red and inflamed, and baby will usually let you know just how uncomfortable he or she feels. Pimples, sores, and blisters may also occur. Strict cleanliness is essential—which means not just frequent diaper changes but frequent rinsing as well. Tight rubber pants or plastic diaper coverings worn for long periods should be avoided. Frequent air drying of the skin is a good idea, and if you use cloth reusable diapers, they should not be laundered in harsh soaps. When the irritation is severe, a doctor should be consulted.

Sunburn

Sunburn is caused by middle-length ultraviolet (UV) rays of the sun—which you do not feel—not by the infrared rays that feel warm on the skin. So you may burn without feeling warm on a cloudy day and feel warm without burning if you take your sun under glass, which screens out the ultraviolet rays but admits the infrared.

Sunburn results in injury to the skin. The skin defends itself by increasing its rate of growth to replace damaged skin, resulting in peeling, and by producing extra melanin (pigment) to screen out further attacks of ultraviolet radiation, which manifests itself as tanning. Chronic exposure to the ultraviolet rays of the sun over the years contributes to early skin wrinkling and to more, larger, and darker liver spots.

It is quite well established that development of skin cancer has direct links to sun exposure. Skin cancer occurs most frequently in fair-skinned people, in people who work in the sun, and in people who play in the sun, and it most often occurs on sun-exposed areas of the skin.

So it is advisable to use sunscreen lotions when you are out in the sun because they block out some ultraviolet light. If your doctor or pharmacist advises that certain medications you are taking will make you more susceptible to sunlight, use a good sunblocker or keep your skin covered. The higher the sun-blocking number that is indicated on the package, the more UV rays are blocked. But remember that lotions quickly wash off with sweating or swimming, and they rub off just by your turning over on a beach blanket. Keep in mind, too, that the sun is highest on June 21 in the Northern Hemisphere (December 21 in the Southern Hemisphere), which means that is when you are exposed to the most direct UV rays. Early sunbathers should be aware that the sun is at the same height in the sky in May as it is in August, which means you can suffer as much sun damage in May as in August despite a little spring chill in the air.

Heat and Chemical Burns

Fire, scalding water, and abrasive chemicals cause direct and instantaneous injury. These burns are classified according to the depth of the injury and the amount of damage to the various skin tissues.

First-Degree Burns

Surface skin is hurt, but living skin cells are not damaged. There is pain, redness, and perhaps some swelling. This burn heals by itself in a few days.

Second-Degree Burns

Here, in addition to pain and redness, there is blistering and weeping of fluid. Living epidermal cells just below the surface skin are killed, but the epidermal layer remains largely intact and will rebuild itself within a month or less without scarring.

Third-Degree Burns

Third-degree burns completely destroy cells of the epidermal layer so that new skin cannot be regenerated at the burn site and scarring will result. The deeper dermal layer and even the fatty tissue underneath may be destroyed. The skin will probably look charred or otherwise eroded. There may not be pain immediately if nerve endings have been destroyed. These are always serious and skin grafting is usually necessary for proper healing.

Because it is not always easy to tell the difference between second- and third-degree burns, even for a physician, any serious burn as large as an inch or more should be shown to a doctor. There is always danger of infection.

When extremely severe burns have been sustained, as when someone has been taken from a burning building or subjected to extensive scalding, you can assume third-degree burns have occurred and expert help should be sought at once. Kitchen burns, when they occur quickly and there is no prolonged contact with a hot surface, flame, superheated fat, or scalding water, are usually first or second degree. Sunburn is generally a first-degree burn, but prolonged exposure of sensitive skin can result in the blistering and swelling of second-degree sunburns. Chemical burns can continue to increase in severity if the irritating substance is not thoroughly flushed away from the skin.

Third-degree burns must be managed with the utmost of expert care, especially if they are extensive. They can be life-threatening. When the skin covering is removed, the body loses fluids in great quantities and it is laid open to the most massive and dangerous infections.

Blisters

The current philosophy is to leave blisters pretty much alone. The skin covering a blister serves to protect the damaged skin underneath while it repairs itself. Cover the blister to protect it from further damage. If the blister has broken by itself, apply an antibiotic ointment (on the drugstore shelf it is usually labeled "triple antibiotic ointment") and cover it with a dry bandage. Extensive blistering from burns or irritants or any sign of infection should be seen by a doctor.

Dry Skin

Everyone knows about dry skin from watching television commercials, and each of us has a favorite remedy for the problem that may range in price from a few cents to many dollars depending on how many "organic" or "natural" ingredients are claimed for the product. But then the earliest records of humankind tell of people anointing themselves with oils, so we must assume that the TV generation is not the first to suffer from dry skin.

Dry skin is dehydration of the surface layer of the skin, which means that water present there naturally has evaporated. Skin tends to be more dry as we age. Domestic and commercial cleaners and solvents remove oils from the skin that help retain moisture, and the skin dries. Wet skin swells and becomes soft while dry skin shrinks and becomes brittle. So when you have your hands in and out of water constantly, the skin may crack and roughen from the continual changes.

Dry skin may be rough and it may peel or flake. There is itching and the consequent scratching makes things worse. Eczema or secondary infection can result from scratching and an itch-scratch cycle can develop.

Treatment for dry skin consists of allowing the water that is naturally present in the skin to stay there. You don't have to "moisturize" your skin—the skin does that by itself. Use an oil to hold in skin moisture (any low-cost hand cream, bath oil, petroleum jelly) and avoid excess soap and other drying agents. If general drying of body skin is a problem, humidifying the atmosphere in winter with a room humidifier will help.

Itching

Sometimes the cause of itching is obvious; sometimes it is not. Chemical irritants, dryness, sweating, or rough clothing can all cause itching. Sensitivity to certain foods or drugs and some systemic diseases cause itching. The list is endless. Rapid temperature changes can cause skin to itch, and nervousness, puzzlement, or confusion can start an itch going. If you are bothered with itching it may get worse at night in a warm bed when you have more time to think about it.

The natural response to itching is rubbing or scratching. Persistent rubbing and scratching can cause a dermatitis that requires more scratching and the itch-scratch cycle begins. In some cases the itch-scratch cycle is so severe that an angry infection results.

Careful inquiry and detective work is usually needed to find the cause of itching when the reason is not obvious, and this is one of those times when a well-kept medical history can pay off. Records of medicines, diet, chronic disorders, lifestyle, and temperament may all provide clues for your doctor.

Localized itches can sometimes be relieved by over-the-counter itch preparations. A 1 percent hydrocortisone ointment is often effective, but it shouldn't be used continuously for more than a week. Using it longer than a week can cause the skin to become thin and fragile for a long time afterward, hindering healing of any condition that may exist. If itching persists, consult your doctor.

Hives

A temporary swelling in the dermal layer of the skin results in a hive—which is sort of a giant mosquito bite, but it is much larger and often irregularly shaped. The swelling is often caused by a histamine, a protein released in response to sensitivity or allergy to some substance. Finding the allergy or source of sensitivity can involve a bit of detective work or the cause may be obvious—an insect bite, a drug just taken, or the observation that hives occur every time you eat a certain food. Stress and nervousness seem to bring them out on some people. When hives are severe, an antihistamine may be prescribed to combat the histamines present. If the onset of hives follows taking a prescribed drug, the doctor should be informed at once because it may herald a more serious reaction later.

Hives may signal a life-threatening situation that is about to happen, especially if they follow an insect bite or taking medicine or eating food a person is known to be allergic to. Hives spreading over the body or general swelling of any body part is a danger signal, and medical help should be sought at once. The danger is that there can be a swelling of the larynx to such a degree that breathing becomes impossible and death can follow quickly. People who know they have severe allergic reactions, to bee or wasp stings, for example, should carry an EpiPen—an injector tube that delivers a single dose of epinephrine.

Outdoor workers and campers who are allergic to bee stings and people who have severe allergic reactions to certain foods should have an EpiPen with them all the time because severe, life-threatening swelling can happen in minutes, long before emergency help can arrive. When exposed to a bee or wasp sting, the allergic person jabs the pen into a thigh muscle (according to instructions in the box that should be read and remembered long before an incident occurs), and it delivers the epinephrine automatically. But emergency medical help is still required; the EpiPen dose is only stopgap first aid.

Contact Dermatitis

This is a skin eruption caused by some irritant—industrial chemicals or poison ivy, for example. If you are allergic or sensitive to a substance with which you come in contact, an eczema can develop within one to three days.

Once again a careful history and a bit of detective work is needed to discover and remove the offending substance. Were you out-of-doors and exposed to poison ivy in the past few days? What other substances have you been exposed to? The site of the irritation may be revealing. Eczema on the wrist or finger may identify a watch, bracelet, or ring as the culprit (even if the jewelry is of a high-karat gold). Blisters in streaky lines on arms or legs point to poison ivy because the plant's irritating oil tends to streak across the skin as you brush against it.

If the contact dermatitis is severe, it is a problem for the special skills of a dermatologist.

Eczema and Dermatitis

The words *eczema* and *dermatitis* are very general words used to refer to many kinds of skin ailments. Eczema describes a series of events that occur on the skin: redness, swelling, the appearance of small, fluid-filled vesicles (tiny blisters), oozing, scaling, and crusting. Dermatitis simply means an inflammation of the skin. To say that you have dermatitis simply means that you have a skin irritation of some kind that has not yet been described precisely. To say that you have eczema means that the skin has gotten a bit messy-looking as a result of something that is wrong with it. There are many causes of eczema and dermatitis, some of which are well known and others that are unknown and puzzling. Following are some of the most common that you are liable to see.

Acne Vulgaris

The pimples, blackheads, nodules, cysts, and scars of acne are too well known to need describing. They occur on the face, neck, shoulders, and back, and when it occurs acne seems to be a body response to hormone changes during puberty. Arising in the teen years it may persist into the late twenties or even the thirties. It is one of the many skin ailments that are poorly understood. The term *vulgaris* added to the medical name is simply a Latin term that means it is a very common form of acne, not vulgar in the sense that we commonly use the word.

It is known that acne is not caused by dirty habits, masturbation, chocolate, greasy foods, or any other identifiable teenage indulgence. On the other hand, it is also known that parental pressure, guilt feelings, social self-consciousness, stress, and tension may precipitate flare-ups.

While the cause of acne is unknown and there is neither cure nor preventive at this time, tremendous strides have been made in treating acne so that improvement in one's appearance can be attained in nearly every case. But acne sufferers should be under the care of a competent dermatologist because a carefully managed program of antibiotics and skin care is often required. Unsupervised home treatment is usually worse than useless. Denying a young person access to care by a competent dermatologist on the assumption that he or she will "outgrow it" is cruel and can lead to scarring of both the skin and the young person's personality that could have been prevented.

Seborrheic Dermatitis

This is yet another dermatitis of unknown cause. Seborrheic dermatitis appears as a red, scaly eruption in the same areas as acne—face, chest, and back—and in addition may invade the scalp. It may first appear in infancy, then disappear, and then return again after puberty and persist all during adult life.

Like so many skin disorders, emotional stress seems to play some mysterious role in recurrences. Dermatologists can treat the symptoms with some success and bring relief to those affected, but there is no cure at the present time.

Psoriasis

Approximately six million people in the United States have psoriasis. No one suffering from psoriasis should restrict him- or herself to patent preparations but should seek professional help. While psoriasis cannot be cured, under the direction of a good dermatologist it is eminently treatable; lesions can be reduced and flare-ups can be minimized.

Psoriasis manifests itself as clusters of slightly raised, scablike plaques that occur most often in bony places such as the knees and elbows. The lesions can occur anywhere on the body, however, and when they are widespread, they can be both demoralizing and debilitating.

Hand Eczemas

Both at home and in the industrial world, hand eczema is the most common skin ailment. When your hands are constantly exposed to drying and irritating agents, as they are in homemaking and many other occupations, some or all of the events that take the name eczema can occur—redness, swelling, the appearance of tiny blisters, oozing, scaling, and crusting. For want of better names, hand eczemas may be designated as dishpan hands, bartender's hands, laboratory hands, and so on, depending on the source of the irritation. Diagnosis is usually made by taking a careful history and conducting laboratory tests to eliminate other possible causes of the eczema.

Heat Rash, or Prickly Heat

This happens when sweat ducts become obstructed. Look for redness and a rash composed of tiny red bumps or small blisters. The condition and the rash become worse with sweating. Looking at the skin with a magnifying glass, you will find that the little bumps or blisters are at sweat pores but never at a pore where there is a hair growing. Anything that helps prevent sweating is helpful—air-conditioning, well-ventilated clothing, and so on.

Pityriasis Rosea

This is yet another skin disorder of unknown cause or origin. (Doctors say "A disease of uncertain etiology," which means "We haven't cracked this one yet.") And, as you may have noticed, there are many of these in the realm of dermatology. This mysterious ailment, however, disappears by itself within about eight weeks as mysteriously as it appears.

Pityriasis rosea is a rash consisting of small pink or red circles that have a collar of scales around the edge. The center of the lesion may be clear or just a bit crinkly or wrinkled. The rash often has a characteristic distribution of arching lines that go from the ears to the hips, and when viewed from the back with some imagination, the pattern may seem to form a crude picture of a fir tree—a Christmas tree. It is often preceded by a "herald patch" or blotch elsewhere on the body.

Diagnosis is usually made by seeing what the lesions look like under a magnifying glass, by observing the fir-tree distribution of lesions, and by the fact that other tests performed by the doctor prove negative.

Skin Infections

The skin is alive with microorganisms—bacteria, viruses, yeasts, and fungi. Sometimes, under certain circumstances, there are small animals such as mites and insects. Most of this wildlife lives on the skin because it is a hospitable environment with plenty of moisture and warmth, innumerable cracks and crannies to hide in, and lots of food in the form of dead skin and body excretions. Practically all these organisms are harmless and some actually help us by keeping down populations of potentially harmful bacteria.

Some villains, however, will invade the skin or even invade the body *through* the skin when they get an opportunity. These cause a variety of infections. Following are some of the most common.

Boils

Most people have experienced boils on occasion, but some people are apparently susceptible to them and get them rather often. A boil is a local infection caused by a staphylococcus bacterium and may arise anywhere on the body; a sty, for example, is a boil on the eyelid.

A boil starts out as a red bump that enlarges slowly until it is as much as ½ inch or even 1½ inches across. There is often throbbing pain or burning. After several days the boil becomes soft and pus-filled. A yellow or white head appears in the middle of its surface. If left alone it will eventually rupture, drain itself of a mixture of pus and blood, and begin to heal.

It is best to have a boil seen and treated by a doctor, especially if it is large, if you get them frequently, or if several appear at the same time. Puncturing or squeezing a boil while it is still hard may make the infection worse. Once the boil is draining, it should be kept clean and covered with a dressing. The staphylococcus bacteria are highly infectious, so until the boil heals, scrupulous cleanliness and careful disposal of dressings should be rigorously enforced.

Medically, a boil is called a furuncle. A carbuncle is several furuncles that connect with each other in the dermal layer of the skin and in the fatty subcutaneous tissue. These are large and painful areas that may persist for as much as two weeks before coming to a head. There may be some fever with carbuncles. They should always be seen and treated by a physician and never treated with home remedies.

Impetigo

This is usually thought of as a disease of small children, and indeed it is seen most frequently among infants and youngsters, but anyone can get impetigo. Once again, streptococcus and staphylococcus bacteria are usually the culprits.

Impetigo starts with a flat area of redness and then tiny blisters develop that break, ooze, and form a brown or yellow crust. It may go away by itself eventually, but spreading and complications are most often the rule if professional help is not sought promptly.

Ringworm

Ringworm is not a worm but a fungal infection whose lesions are roughly ring-shaped. These fungi have a special taste for dead skin, hair, and nails—it's all they eat. Poor hygiene and poor living conditions increase the chances of contracting ringworm, but anyone can get it.

Ringworm of the body is usually flat, scaly, and red. The center of the ring clears as the scaly red edge advances. Ringworm of the scalp produces round, sharply outlined areas where hairs are broken off just above the skin. The lesions may be light and flaky, but they may also be moist and badly inflamed. Both body and scalp ringworm are most common in children and may become epidemic among children who congregate together.

Ringworm of the feet (athlete's foot) affects at least half the adults in the United States at some time during their lives. The fungus is found anywhere that feet go. It causes minor scaling and cracking between the toes, but if left unattended it can spread widely and become badly inflamed. Then, secondary infection can occur. Ringworm of the groin (jock itch) occurs most often in men and may be carried to the groin from affected feet.

Any infection of ringworm should be seen by a doctor so that both the disease and the specific organism causing it can be positively identified and proper treatment prescribed.

Warts

Most people are familiar with these rough, flesh-colored bumps that frequently turn up on the hands. And anyone who has read *Tom Sawyer* knows how to cure warts: You stick the hand with the warts in water gathered in an old stump and say, "Spunk water, spunk water, swallow these warts."

The funny thing about warts is that this and a hundred other folklore remedies often work in getting rid of them even though it has been clearly established that warts are caused by a virus. Wrapping the wart in duct tape can make it disappear in four to six weeks. Over-the-counter preparations found in drugstores also work. The point is that warts seem to be psychosuggestible for reasons that are not yet understood. In laboratory experiments doctors have "cured" warts with treatments as bizarre and as obviously worthless as spunk water. And, using suggestion, they have been able to make a patient's warts disappear on one hand and remain on the other. Warts may also disappear without treatment and without suggestion.

There are, however, many simple and reliable medical cures for warts, so your best bet in dealing with them is to show them to a doctor, especially if you have many of them or get them frequently.

Warts have different names and slightly different appearances depending on where they occur: Finger warts are generally flesh-colored and rough and may have black dots scattered through them. Face, neck, or shoulder warts may be shaped like little fingers. Plantar warts grow on the bottom of the foot and tend to grow inward because of the pressure of standing and walking on them. They can become quite painful. Soft, nonhorny warts that look something like tiny cauliflowers may appear in moist areas—the armpits, groin, anus, and vagina. These are sometimes called venereal warts although they can be acquired in other ways besides sexual contact.

Some people are tempted to pare a wart with a knife or razor blade in an effort to reduce it. This is a bad idea for any blood from the wart will contain live virus that can spread the wart to other sites nearby. If a wart has to be removed quickly for cosmetic reasons, freezing or electrocautery, performed by a physician, is usually effective.

Herpes Simplex

The herpes simplex virus is best known for causing fever blisters (cold sores) about the mouth, but it may invade the skin anywhere or the mucous membranes inside the mouth, the eyes, or the genitals, where it can produce angry infections.

Herpes simplex skin infections usually show up as clusters of tiny blisters that may be mixed with pimples. These ooze and form crusts, and there is often swelling and redness. On mucous membranes of the mouth or genitals, herpes simplex appears as a cluster of pitted sores surrounded by a red, inflamed-looking area. Herpes infections around the eyes can endanger eyesight and should be seen by a doctor at once.

Herpes infections are recurrent in some people. Fever blisters about the mouth, for example, may come and go at the same site several times a year. There is no preventive and no known cure at this time, but if an infection is extensive or painful, symptoms should be treated by a doctor to bring as much relief as possible and to avoid secondary infections. Acyclovir and famciclovir are two antiviral medications a doctor may prescribe for people whose outbreaks of herpes are frequent and troublesome.

Herpes often blooms in susceptible people in times of high stress, and sun exposure will bring out sores in others. Obviously, then, reducing stress and using sunblockers can help. The herpes virus that causes cold sores is not the same as the herpes virus that causes genital herpes. They are the same family of villains, but they are not identical, and herpes from a cold sore doesn't cause genital herpes.

Shingles

Shingles is caused by the herpes zoster virus, the same virus that causes chicken pox, and it is thought that after a case of chicken pox the virus may lie dormant for years and somehow become reactivated. Shingles appears as a rash of small blisters running in a line from back to front around the chest, abdomen, neck, or face following nerve pathways. It usually appears only on one side of the body. If it appears on the head and affects the eye, it is a particularly serious problem that requires immediate consultation with an ophthalmologist.

There may be substantial pain with shingles called postherpetic neuralgia. If this occurs, the doctor can usually shorten the time that pain persists using the antiviral medications mentioned previously, acyclovir or famciclovir.

Canker Sores

Canker sores occur only in the mucous membrane lining of the mouth. They are similar in appearance to herpes simplex, but they are not caused by the herpes virus. It is not known, in fact, what causes canker sores, and there is no treatment except to alleviate pain and try to prevent secondary infections. The sores heal in a week or ten days, and they tend to recur at the same sites in people who get them. Dentists working with college students have reported seeing small epidemics of canker sores that coincide with exam time.

Skin Ulcers

A skin ulcer might better be called a nasty-looking sore. Ulcers result from causes as obvious as an injury, or they may result from something more obscure, such as poor circulation in the legs, diabetes, a malignancy, or syphilis.

If a skin ulcer appears that can't be explained by an injury, or if a sore persists and becomes worse instead of healing quickly, it should be shown to a doctor without delay. If a painless ulcer appears in the groin area (especially on the genitals), on the mouth or tongue, or on the breast or nipples, syphilis may be suspected as a possible cause. (A more detailed discussion of the signs of syphilis can be found in one of the following sections where we discuss systemic disorders that show on the skin.)

Ulcers that appear on the lower parts of the legs, on the ankles or feet, and that persist or recur are usually caused by poor circulation in the veins or arteries. This is most often seen in older people. The sore is likely to begin as a painful red spot that becomes blue or purplish. The skin then breaks down to form an ulcer.

Lice and Scabies

While the infections we have been talking about are caused by invading microorganisms, lice and scabies are infestations of small parasitic insects. Lice are tiny, bloodsucking insects, while scabies are even tinier, spider-like animals that burrow under the skin.

Lice live on body hairs or in clothing and venture forth from time to time to get a meal of blood. Itching is severe and eggs and developing lice can be found attached to a hair or a thread of clothing.

Crab lice are a variety of body lice that inhabit the pubic area. They are smaller than body lice and are harder to see with the naked eye. Under a magnifying glass they are seen to have little pincers that make them look like crabs—hence their name.

In scabies, the female mite burrows under the skin to lay eggs. There is severe itching, often just at bedtime, and you can see red lines on the skin where the mite has done its burrowing. The doctor will treat both lice and scabies by prescribing a pesticide and will check for any infection that may have been caused by scratching. Then, clothing and bedclothes must be scrupulously laundered.

Caution: All skin infections should be handled cautiously to prevent spreading the infection to others or to other parts of the body. Extra-special care should be taken not to transfer microorganisms from a skin infection to a skin area that is injured (scratched, for example) or already raw from another ailment.

Most skin ailments are not contagious, however, and it is quite disturbing psychologically for a person with a noninfectious skin ailment to have others shrink away. Acne is not contagious, and neither are psoriasis or vitiligo. People with these ailments

should be given the reassurance of touching by their families.

Systemic Diseases That Show on the Skin

A number of ailments that affect the body systems—and so are usually called systemic diseases—may affect the skin as well. People in good health, especially children, have an unmistakable glow about them that bespeaks their well-being. Pallor, flushing, dryness, unreasonable sweating, rashes—all speak of something wrong going on inside that should be investigated.

When a systemic disease is present, such as measles, scarlet fever, or chicken pox, there is first a general feeling of malaise, fever, and so on, and then a characteristic rash appears on the skin. Skin lesions are the only outward signs of the presence of early syphilis. Drugs you are allergic to may cause skin eruptions. Following are brief descriptions of some common systemic ailments that show themselves on the skin.

Syphilis

The corkscrew-shaped spirochete that causes syphilis can penetrate intact, healthy skin, and within hours it enters the bloodstream. So syphilis can be said to be a systemic disease from the outset.

In a little more than a week or as much as a month after the initial infection, one sore, called a chancre, will appear on the skin at the site where the spirochetes entered—on the genitals, mouth parts, or elsewhere depending on how sexual contact was made with the affected partner. And, incidentally, it may not be obvious that a partner has syphilis in an infectious stage.

The chancre is painless, round, and slightly raised and has a hard base that may feel as if there is a nickel or a dime buried under the skin. Left alone, the chancre will heal in thirty to ninety days, but the spirochetes remain and continue to multiply and circulate in the bloodstream. This is primary syphilis.

The next episode, secondary syphilis, results from a systemwide reaction to the spirochete. This appears on the skin as a generalized rash involving all skin surfaces, even the palms of the hands and the soles of the feet and the mucous lining of the mouth. The nature of the rash may vary from one individual to the next, but an identifying feature is that all skin marks appear the same— all red and flat, all raised and scaly, all red bumps, and so on. Whenever a doctor sees a generalized, uniform rash that shows lesions on the palms and soles, he or she suspects syphilis until it can be proved otherwise through blood tests.

The rash, too, disappears and the syphilis becomes latent for a number of years. When it next turns up, it may affect any part of the body. Some favorite sites are the central nervous system, the heart, and the arteries leading to the heart.

The greatest danger from syphilis comes from ignoring early symptoms because they are painless and disappear spontaneously. It is a most serious disease at any stage, and even a suspicion that it exists should be enough to send you to a physician for diagnosis and treatment if necessary.

Drug Eruption

When any skin eruption—rash, redness, hives, or whatever—appears while you are taking any drug, even aspirin, the drug should be suspected as one possible cause of the skin problem. And when drugs are suspected, the person's general condition should be monitored carefully on the chance that the skin eruption is heralding a more serious allergic reaction. If a doctor has prescribed the drug, he or she should be notified at once of the reaction.

Measles, Chicken Pox, and Scarlet Fever

Measles is a serious disease and too often a deadly one. Fortunately, most children in developed countries are now routinely immunized against this disease so it is not seen nearly so much as it once was. If measles does appear, however, a doctor should always be consulted.

The measles rash is purplish-red and as a general rule first appears in the head area— on the forehead, behind the ears, and on the neck. It then spreads to involve the whole body. The small spots are flat (not raised) and as new ones appear farther down the body, the old ones tend to merge together to become big, splashy spots. A cough may precede the appearance of spots on the skin, and if the throat is examined at this time, you may see tiny white spots inside the cheeks. These are called Koplik's spots.

To look for Koplik's spots, peer into the mouth using a flashlight. Gently drag a wooden tongue blade or the edge of a teaspoon across the inside of the cheek from back to front. As you scrape away the saliva from inside the cheek, you should see the white spots if they are there.

German measles (rubella) is the infamous villain that produces birth defects when a pregnant woman contracts the disease. It is important, therefore, for women of childbearing age to know if they have had the disease and have thus been rendered immune to subsequent attacks. This information should be a part of the personal health record.

The onset of German measles may be heralded by a fever, a feeling of illness, and a swelling of lymph nodes behind the ears and at the base of the skull. The rash differs from measles in that, after appearing on the face or chest, it spreads quickly over the body in a day or so. Old spots disappear as new ones turn up farther down the body. The whole process takes only two or three days, while measles rash lasts at least a week.

If suspected, the presence of German measles should be confirmed by a doctor even if the ailment seems superficial. Then a positive record can be made for future reference. Immunization against mumps, measles, and rubella (MMR) is routinely administered to infants. This, too, should be entered in a permanent health record.

Chicken pox, like the others, is preceded by illness and fever. While children usually get along with chicken pox tolerably well, adults may become severely ill. In any event, and despite its innocuous name, chicken pox should be seen by a doctor.

Red dots and then blisters appear on the trunk of the body. These blisters break and get crusty, and some may become pus-filled. Itching is likely to be severe. The illness will last a week or ten days and then the spots and sores will take somewhat longer to disappear.

Scarlet fever is a streptococcal infection that can lead to serious complications if left untreated; so a physician should always be consulted when it is suspected.

Scarlet fever is easy to confuse with measles at the outset, with the rash starting out as a redness about the neck and spreading to the rest of the body. The difference is that many dot-sized eruptions cover a bright red skin, making the skin feel rough. The face is flushed except for a rather obvious area around the mouth, which is a characteristic identifying mark of the disease. Peeling, similar to that caused by sunburn, occurs as the rash subsides.

Nervous, Emotional, or Psychological Skin Responses

One of the most mysterious and fascinating aspects of human skin is the way it is affected by the emotions, stress, or tension. When you consider how fear, joy, embarrassment, and other emotions are reflected in skin changes, it is not hard to believe that skin ailments may be affected by the emotions as well. It seems to be true, but it is still a facet of skin studies that is not at all understood by dermatologists.

We have seen how warts may appear to come and go at will or can be gotten rid of at times by psychic suggestion even though they are caused by a virus. The virus herpes simplex may live in the body for years and then suddenly cause a fever blister during a time of tension or upset. Flare-ups of acne, psoriasis, canker sores, and many other skin ailments have been seen to occur in patients under emotional stress. A rash, severe itching, or hives may occur with no better explanation than "nervousness" and

may disappear mysteriously when the patient is told of the probable psychic cause of the ailment.

All this is not to say that a skin ailment should be ignored with the assumption, or the hope, that it is only "imagined" and will go away when one sets his or her thoughts straight. Far from it. Skin ailments should be seen by a professional, and the source of the ailment should be scientifically established if at all possible. Then the sufferer should be given emotional support and reassurance as well as medication, which is good therapy when dealing with any bodily ill.

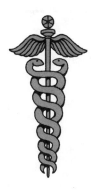

10

Tests and Observations of the Reproductive Organs

Despite the deluge of revealing surveys and reports on human sexuality that have appeared during the past thirty years, it is still easier to find an honest politician than it is to find someone with an accurate knowledge of his or her reproductive organs. Most people have only the vaguest notion of how the reproductive systems work and just the sketchiest ideas of what equipment exists "down there," what it does, and what can go wrong.

Like other systems of the body, the reproductive systems are susceptible to a number of ailments. Unfortunately, the aura of mystery that surrounds the reproductive organs induces many people either to overestimate their problems or to turn a blind and embarrassed eye on signs of real trouble. This combination of misinformation and embarrassment exacts a high toll in death and disability, especially among women. Cancers of the breast, cervix, and uterus—in which cure rates run better than 80 percent with early detection—together are the

leading cause of death among women in their thirties and forties. And venereal disease continues as a major social scourge despite years of effort at public education.

The procedure for tracking the health of your reproductive system is the same as it is for the other body systems: You should know what organs are involved, where they are, and what they do; you should know what feels right and looks right for you when the system is functioning normally; and there are some basic tests and critical observations you should make to spot early signs of trouble or to reassure yourself that all is going well.

The Female External Genital Organs

The outer genital organs are collectively called the vulva, and this includes the whole area between the legs except for the anus. There is no reason why you can't examine this entire area if you want to, except that it

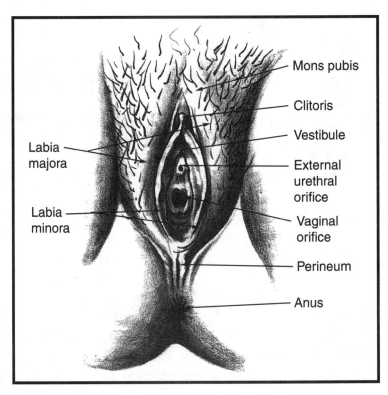

Female External Genital Area

takes a bit of arranging and a fair amount of flexibility. Most women feel that the lessons learned are well worth the effort, however. If you elect to try, you will need a medium-sized mirror and a good light source to illuminate the area you are inspecting. Sit on the floor with your knees bent and spread apart, and arrange the mirror and light to get the best view possible. It's not an ideal way to conduct an examination, but it's the best you can do.

Beginning at the front, the most prominent feature is the mons pubis, a pad of fatty tissue covering the pubic bone. This is the triangular area that is covered with pubic hair. The labia majora, the fleshy outer lips of the genitals, separate from the mons and proceed backward surrounding the outer organs and openings. Immediately below the mons pubis is the clitoris, a tiny piece of very sensitive tis-

sue, analogous in some ways to the male penis; it is largely made of erectile tissue, as the penis is, and both organs arise from the same site in a developing fetus. The difference is, of course, that the clitoris does not contain the urethra, the tube leading from the urinary bladder, and the penis does.

The clitoris is partially hidden by the upper end of the labia minora, two thin folds of skin that follow along inside the labia majora. These form a hood over the clitoris in the front and surround the urethral opening and the vaginal opening in an area called the vestibule. The urethra can be seen as a small protrusion just forward of the larger vaginal opening. You may also be able to see the hymen or its vestiges, a bit of membranous tissue that partially obstructs the lower end of the vagina. In a self-examination, this irregular fringe of tissue is sometimes mistaken for small growths, which it is not. The anus, the end of the digestive tract, is the obvious opening behind the vulva and is separated from it by an area known as the perineum.

The Female Internal Genital Organs

The vagina is a thin-walled muscular tube whose lower opening we have just described in the vestibule of the vulva. It proceeds upward for about four inches until it meets the cervix, which is the opening into the uterus, or womb. The uterus is located just behind and above the bladder and in front of the rectum, which puts it just about in the middle of the body. If you draw a line around your body at about the level where bikini pants come, you will be pretty much in the plane of the uterus. Because a pregnancy shows somewhat higher than this, most people believe that the resting uterus is higher than it actually is.

The uterus is not very large—only about the size of a small fist. The walls are relatively thick and muscular and the interior cavity is hardly more than a slit until it begins to

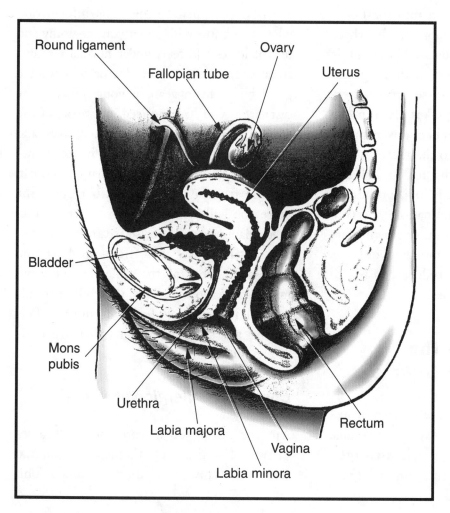

Round ligament

Fallopian tube

Ovary

Uterus

Bladder

Mons pubis

Urethra

Labia majora

Vagina

Labia minora

Rectum

Female Internal Reproductive Organs

expand to accommodate a growing fetus. Then the walls thicken and the internal cavity of the uterus expands dramatically. Extending outward from either side of the upper end of the uterus are the fallopian tubes, each of which is about four inches long. The ends of these tubes flare out, like the horn of a trumpet, and nestled in the shadow of each horn is an ovary about the size of a walnut.

The ovaries produce two female sex hormones, estrogen and progesterone, which encourage development of the female sex characteristics and regulate the menstrual cycle. In addition, each month one of the ovaries releases a mature egg. This is called ovulation. The egg is drawn into the horn-shaped end of the nearby fallopian tube where it makes its way to the uterus. If the egg is not fertilized along the way, it disintegrates and is disposed of in vaginal secretions. Fertilization of a mature egg takes place in one of the fallopian tubes. When this happens the fertilized egg moves to the uterus where it becomes implanted in the uterine wall and begins to grow. When the fallopian tubes are blocked because of inflammation, scarring from disease, or for some other reason, fertilization can't take place and the woman is sterile. A sterilization procedure consists of tying off the fallopian tubes.

Trouble Signs in the External Genital Organs

The woman does not exist who has not had distress signals from her external genitals. These signals include unusual discharges, itching, burning, chafing, and pain in degrees ranging from petty annoyance to major discomfort. Sometimes lesions appear: sores, blisters, rashes, lumps, bumps, and so on.

No unusual sign or signal from the vulval region should be ignored if it persists for more than a few days. You should not suffer stoically or embarrassedly waiting for itching or an abnormal discharge to "go away." Many rampaging and damaging infections can get a head start on you while you wait for them to cure themselves. A doctor should be consulted. As with any other complaint, the doctor will want as much information as you can give: the exact location of the problem, how it feels, how long you have been having trouble, and so on. You are best equipped to give this information when you know a bit about your anatomy and how it looks and feels under normal circumstances. In addition, the doctor will want a good bit of history about your periods, any discharges you have noticed, what sort of life you lead, what type of contraceptives and douches you use, and even what kind of clothes you wear. And the more information you can provide from a personal health record, the more you will help the doctor to arrive at an exact diagnosis and precise treatment.

Self-diagnosis is difficult at best and impossible most of the time, but you can make some observations that will provide helpful information for your doctor. Following are some conditions that are definitely abnormal.

Contact or Allergic Vulvitis

An *-itis* ending on a word means "inflammation of"—thus vulvitis means inflammation of the vulva, the external genitals. This area can become inflamed as a result of direct contact with an irritating agent or as an allergic reaction to a substance taken internally. Women with sensitive skin may suffer a vulvar reaction as a result of contact with such seemingly innocent materials as perfumed toilet paper, bubble-bath products, douche ingredients, feminine spray deodorants, a new bath soap, or new synthetic fabrics in undergarments—especially in tight bikini pants. Similarly, vulvitis has also been diagnosed as an allergic reaction to common medications such as aspirin, sulfa drugs, and some laxatives.

Vulvitis is indicated by a reddening of the vulvar skin accompanied by itching. In more severe cases the inner and outer vaginal lips may become swollen, and clear, bubblelike blisters may erupt. These will eventually drain and crust over.

Treatment consists of identifying the culprit and avoiding contact with it in the future. This is largely a trial-and-error process in which you identify recent changes in personal hygiene—new underwear, the use of deodorized tampons, perfumed douches, or contraceptive foams, or new medications, including both over-the-counter and prescription drugs. Then, you eliminate them one by one until you notice an improvement in your condition. Meanwhile, your doctor can confirm the diagnosis of vulvitis and can prescribe soothing preparations to alleviate the more severe symptoms.

Enlarged Bartholin's Glands

Bartholin's glands are two small, mucous-producing glands located within the vestibule formed by the labia minora on either side of the vaginal opening. They provide natural lubrication during intercourse. Normally you can neither see nor feel them. Occasionally, however, one or both of these glands can become blocked and subsequently infected, creating painful, pus-filled cysts.

You can check for Bartholin's cysts by gently rolling the inner lips, or labia minora, on either side of the vaginal opening between your thumb and forefinger. A noticeable swelling that is tender to the touch is likely to be an enlarged Bartholin's gland and should be treated by your doctor. The pain, however, is likely to send you to the doctor before you bother to check yourself.

Genital Warts

Like warts elsewhere on the body, genital warts are caused by a virus. While they seem to be most commonly transmitted through sexual intercourse with an infected person, they can be acquired by other means as well.

In their early stages, genital warts are small, pinkish-tan growths not much bigger than grains of rice. You may find two or three around the vaginal opening or small clusters along the labia. They thrive on vaginal secretions, discharges, and moisture and can be spread to other areas of the vulva by scratching. Once they have gained a foothold, genital warts can mushroom into large, cauliflowerlike masses. In extreme cases, they can interfere with intercourse, urination, and defecation.

Having a Pap smear every six months after finding genital warts is recommended because of a suspected link with cervical cancer.

Gonorrhea

Gonorrhea is one of the most prevalent communicable diseases in the United States. However, most women infected with gonorrhea don't even know they have it. In fact, 80 percent will be completely asymptomatic—that is, free of overt symptoms that would alert them to the presence of this venereal disease. But as the bacteria that causes gonorrhea works its way up the vagina, through the cervix and into the uterus, the disease can spread to the fallopian tubes, resulting in scarring of the tubes and permanent sterility.

Early symptoms of gonorrhea in women, when they occur, include burning and frequent urination, which may be mistaken for a passing bladder infection, and a thick greenish-yellow discharge that is almost impossible to distinguish from nonvenereal discharges without a culture test. A culture test involves smearing a sample of the discharge on a special culture plate that encourages the growth of the gonococcus bacteria, incubating it for a period of time, and then examining the culture for characteristic signs indicating the presence of *Neisseria gonorrhoeae*.

Traditionally, this test has been performed almost exclusively in medical laboratories by technicians who prepare a culture and interpret the results of specimens sent to them by doctors. In recent years, however, medical manufacturers have developed a diagnostic test for gonorrhea that can be performed by a doctor or informed assistant in the doctor's office and does not have to be sent out to a laboratory. With medical self-help becoming more and more popular,

it is highly possible that one day such kits will become available at the corner drugstore along with the currently popular urine and pregnancy tests.

Syphilis

The confirming test for syphilis is a blood test that must be performed by a doctor or medical laboratory. If you suspect you may have been exposed to syphilis and you can't or don't want to contact a local doctor, call your state department of health or the U.S. Public Health Service, or walk into any hospital with an emergency receiving division and explain your problem.

Even the vaguest suspicion that a sexual partner may have been infected should be enough to cause you to have a blood test. And a suspicion is all you may have until symptoms become manifest, because infectious syphilis in a partner is rarely obvious. Then, your own symptoms may come and go with minimum discomfort so that you can be lulled into complacency until it is too late for successful treatment.

If you have been exposed to syphilis within the last nine to ninety days, your examination of the vulva may reveal a single, painless sore known as a chancre. This represents the site where the corkscrew-shaped spirochete that causes syphilis entered your body. The chancre is painless, round, and slightly raised and has a hard base that may feel as if there is a nickel or a dime buried under the skin. A syphilitic chancre is commonly accompanied by painless, hard, swollen lymph nodes in the area of the groin. If the chancre is hidden within the vaginal canal, you may miss it in a casual examination.

While the spirochete may penetrate any skin area or mucous membrane—such as the lips, tongue, and tonsils—its most common site of entry is the genital area. You should thoroughly inspect the inner and outer lips of the vagina for this characteristic sore. Left alone, the chancre will heal in thirty to ninety days, but the spirochetes remain and continue to multiply and circulate in the bloodstream. The secondary stage of syphilis is indicated by a generalized skin rash that appears anywhere from a few days to a few weeks after the chancre heals. (For a more detailed description of the rash of secondary syphilis, see Chapter 9 on the skin.) Left untreated, the disease will proceed to invade other organs, the heart and brain being among the favored sites.

Genital Herpes

Genital herpes is a disease caused by contact with the herpes simplex virus. There are actually two strains of this virus. The first, called herpes simplex type I, is responsible for the common cold sore and fever blister around the mouth and lips. A second, related strain, referred to as herpes simplex type II, affects the vulva, the upper vagina, and the cervix.

If either partner in sexual contact has an active herpetic lesion on the genitalia—an open sore like a cold sore—the herpes can be transmitted from one partner to the other. Abstinence during a herpes outbreak is advisable. Using a condom is next best.

Genital herpes is indicated by the presence of small, raised blisters along the vulva and the genital mucous membrane. In the course of a typical episode, which lasts from two to three weeks, the blisters develop into open sores with little holes in them; these become crusted, scabbed over, and, finally, runny. This skin complaint can cause intense itching and distress and is usually accompanied by fever, swollen and painful lymph nodes in the groin area, and an overall run-down feeling. While the acute symptoms disappear when the infection has run its course, the virus continues to be harbored in the body and can flare up again without warning. Subsequent episodes of this recurring disease are usually milder than the initial attack.

As you can see, signs of genital herpes may be confused with the symptoms of severe contact or allergic vulvitis. If you have reason to believe you have contracted genital herpes, you should consult your doctor for a positive diagnosis and help in relieving its more distressing symptoms. Some doctors recommend a Pap smear every six months after genital herpes because of a suspected link with cervical cancer.

Avoiding Sexually Transmitted Diseases

Unless a woman is in a proven monogamous relationship and has very good reason to believe that her partner is free of sexually transmitted diseases (STDs), she should insist that a condom be used during sexual intercourse. People are not vaccinated or otherwise immunized against sexually transmitted diseases, so the only preventive is avoiding contact with the causative agents. The condom, while not a foolproof device, is the best general defense we have available.

While it is the man who uses a condom and should feel a responsibility to do so, women should insist that this responsibility is seen to for their own safety.

Keeping Track of the Internal Genital Organs

Like other internal body organs, the internal genitals are best kept track of by observing how they function rather than by trying to examine them. Self-examination of the vagina and the cervix is possible, but it's rather too difficult for most people and the results are unreliable. What is happening when all of the organs of your reproductive system are working together is considerably more important than any single observation you may make with difficulty. As with other body systems, you should observe what is normal for you and then be alert for changes that may signal all is not as it should be. Here are some things to watch for.

The Menstrual Cycle

Menstrual periods should be regular and should not cause undue distress. Many women have a certain amount of pain with periods, but if you are regularly incapacitated before, during, or following a menstrual period, this should be investigated by a gynecologist. If you have had relatively pain-free periods and suddenly have painful ones, you should seek medical advice; something may definitely be wrong.

Any change in the menstrual cycle is clearly an indication for a visit to the doctor. A number of disorders, both of the reproductive system and parts of the body nominally unrelated to the reproductive system, can affect the regularity of menstrual periods. For example, a change in the state of the thyroid gland almost always affects the menstrual cycle.

Vaginal Bleeding

Unexpected vaginal bleeding is an important finding, and when this occurs, medical help should always be sought. Women who are taking birth control pills may have a phenomenon called breakthrough bleeding, which is slight bleeding or spotting between periods. This is generally nothing to be concerned about, but if it happens do two things: Read the literature that comes with your birth control pills to see what it says about unexpected bleeding, then report the situation to your gynecologist to confirm that this is to be expected from your pill prescription.

Some women who still use an intrauterine device (IUD) may find they have unexpected bleeding and, once again, confirm with your doctor that this is normal. If you do not wear an IUD and you are not taking birth control pills, you should not bleed unless you are having a menstrual period. Other bleeding should be investigated professionally at once.

Pain

Because all the internal genital organs are located low in the pelvis, any problems related to these organs will generally center low in the torso, either in front or in back. But because this area also contains many other organs—the bladder, intestines, nerves, muscles, and so on—pain low in the torso is not indicative of any one thing; and if the pain doesn't persist, it may be completely unimportant. But persistent pain anywhere in the body should be investigated.

Except for the first few times, intercourse should not cause pain. If intercourse becomes painful, a physician should be consulted. Several diseases can cause painful intercourse and, as is true with male impotence, some psychological factors can cause painful intercourse as well. A woman should not assume that painful intercourse is a psychological problem, however, especially if she is happily married or has a satisfactory relationship, without first consulting a gynecologist.

Vaginal Discharges

Vaginal discharges are responsible for a wide range of complaints including itching, soreness and burning of the vulva, chafing of the inner thighs, and painful urination.

The mucous membranes that line the vagina secrete a small amount of milky discharge that lubricates the vagina just as saliva lubricates the mouth. Normally, these vaginal secretions have a slightly acidic pH value that kills yeast, fungi, and other harmful organisms. This delicate balance, however, can be upset by a number of factors including disease, an infection in some other part of the body, antibiotics, birth control pills, excessive douching, pregnancy, irritation of the vagina, a poor diet, or lack of sleep, to name just a few. When something happens to disturb the normal acidity of the vagina, other organisms normally held in check can multiply all out of proportion, resulting in an abnormal discharge that irritates the surrounding tissues.

Three of the most common offenders are *Trichomonas vaginalis*, better known as Trich or TV, for short; *Candida albicans*, a fungal infection also called Monilia or just yeast; and *Haemophilus vaginalis*, or HV, a bacterial infection. Diagnosing the exact culprit in a vaginal infection usually requires microscopic examination of the secretions, or a culture, and it is not uncommon to be afflicted by more than one infection at the same time. Generally you should be suspicious of any thick, copious, malodorous discharge that irritates or inflames the vagina or vulva. A good rule to apply to vaginal discharges is that they do not normally cause you discomfort. When they do, you should suspect a vaginal infection and see your doctor for treatment.

Yeast infections are among the more common of the various vaginal infections and can be treated successfully at home with over-the-counter medications that used to be available only by prescription. But if the discharge you are treating persists after one treatment with such a medication, you should see your doctor at once because it is clearly not a yeast infection. The recommended length of treatment varies among the various brands, so it is important to follow the manufacturer's instructions carefully.

When you have a vaginal infection, it is advisable to wear cotton panties, which afford better air circulation than synthetics. Yeast infections are often helped by eating live-culture yogurt and other foods that help increase the acidity of the vagina.

The Pap Smear

A well-managed health-maintenance program for women must include an annual Pap smear. This is not an observation or test you can do yourself, but it is worth discussing for a moment because of its importance as a life-saving technique and because certain misconceptions about what it does seem to persist despite three decades of publicity and education by various health agencies.

Cervical and uterine cancers are the third leading cause of death among women in some age groups. It is a significant killer in all age groups, even among women in their twenties. When the disease is discovered early, however, cure rates for cervical and uterine cancers are extremely high. The purpose of the Pap smear is to discover early the presence of cancer cells in the uterus. Opinions vary among doctors about how often a woman should have a Pap smear, but the majority opinion seems to favor an annual test and it is routinely performed as part of a regular gynecological examination. The word *regular* is the key

term when it comes to detecting potential problems early.

Keep in mind that the Pap smear is only a cancer test, it doesn't test for venereal disease or pregnancy or Monilia or anything else. The test is named for Dr. George Papanicolaou, who invented the staining technique that is needed to study the sample cells under a microscope.

A speculum is inserted into the vagina to expand the canal and permit examination of the vaginal walls and the cervix. The doctor then gently scrapes a few loose surface cells from the cervix with a small wooden or plastic paddle. These cells are immediately smeared on a microscope slide and sprayed with a special fixative. The fixed slide is then sent to a medical laboratory where it is stained to make microscopic examination of the cells possible.

The slides are interpreted as being one of six groups: Class 0 means that the sample is inadequate for diagnosis for some reason; Class 1 means that the cells are entirely normal; Class 2 is negative for cancer but the technician has found some other kinds of abnormal cells that should be looked into; Class 3 means that cancer cells are suspected; Class 4 is positive for cancer; and Class 5 is strongly positive for cancer. Your doctor will let you know if your test is other than Class 1.

Testing for Ovulation

As we pointed out earlier, a single mature egg erupts from one of the ovaries once a month, is caught in the hornlike end of a fallopian tube, and makes its way to the uterus. If the egg is fertilized on the way, a pregnancy begins. If the egg is not fertilized by a male sperm, the egg disintegrates and is disposed of. Thus, a woman is fertile for a very short period every month.

The eruption of an egg from an ovary is called ovulation, and it occurs about fourteen days after the beginning of a menstrual period. Being able to identify the time of ovulation can serve two purposes: If you want to become pregnant, this is the best time for intercourse. If you do not want to become pregnant and you are not using other contraceptive methods, you will want to abstain from intercourse four or five days before you ovulate and a couple of days afterward. This is the basis of the rhythm method of contraception. Because the egg released by the ovary has an active life of about twelve hours and male sperm can survive two or three days after intercourse, if you wish to minimize your chances of becoming pregnant, you can calculate when *not* to have intercourse. What makes the rhythm method unreliable is that menstrual cycles are not always precisely on schedule, and this often throws off the calculations just enough to allow fertilization to occur.

You can purchase any of several ovulation prediction test kits for home use at the drugstore for about $30 or $40. As with all test kits, the manufacturer's instructions have to be followed carefully. Because of the cost you would probably only want to use this kit when you are planning for a pregnancy. If you are tracking for the long haul to try to avoid pregnancy by the rhythm method, you may want to try to identify your ovulation time using your basal body temperature (BBT), a method that requires care and patience.

Your BBT is the temperature of your body at complete rest. This temperature is taken orally immediately upon awakening in the morning and is usually about one and one-half degrees lower than your normal body temperature. If you were to take your BBT each morning, you would notice a slight drop immediately followed by a sharp rise in temperature approximately two weeks from the first day of your menstrual period. This monthly rise in the BBT is triggered by ovulation, which stimulates hormone production. By charting your BBT over a period of months, you can determine when you are ovulating and identify the short period of fertility. It will also show if, indeed, you are ovulating, which is the first thing a doctor will want to know if you are having trouble becoming pregnant when you want to.

Tracking Ovulation Using Basal Body Temperature

You will need a BBT thermometer. This is a special oral thermometer with a scale of 95° to 100° F (35° to 38° C) with widely spaced, tenth-degree gradations that make it easy for you to detect slight variations in temperature. An ordinary fever thermometer will work but will not be so easy to read.

1. Using a sheet of graph paper, prepare a chart of your menstrual cycle. Across the

top of the chart, list the days in your menstrual cycle. The first day of your menstrual period is day #1. If your cycle is normally twenty-eight days long, your chart will be twenty-eight squares across. If your period comes every thirty-one days, your chart will be thirty-one squares across, and so on. Down the left-hand side of the chart, mark degrees in temperature, from 99.0° F down to 96.5° F or lower in tenth-degree gradations.

2. Beginning with the first day of your menstrual flow, start tracking your BBT. Keep your thermometer on your bedside table, and pop it into your mouth first thing in the morning *before* you get out of bed or before you are even fully awake. Be sure it has been properly shaken down the night before so it is ready to use.

3. Record your temperature each day by locating the temperature registered on your thermometer in the left-hand column of your chart, and then follow this line across until you come to the square under the appropriate day of your cycle. Make a little *x* at this spot.

4. At the end of your cycle, draw a line connecting the *x*'s you have charted. Repeat this procedure for three or four months. You now have a graphic depiction of your ovulatory cycle.

5. If you are ovulating, you will notice a drop immediately followed by a sharp rise of between 0.5° and 1.0° F in your

BBT. This will happen around the fourteenth day of each cycle. The low point represents the time of ovulation. When your temperature goes back up it will stay there, with slight variations, until two or three days prior to the onset of your next menstrual period, at which point your BBT drops and a new cycle begins. If you fail to ovulate in any given cycle, your BBT will not vary by more than two- or three-tenths of a degree for the whole cycle. If, on the other hand, you ovulate and the egg is fertilized, your BBT will remain elevated. This is one of the earliest signs of a possible pregnancy.

Do-It-Yourself Pregnancy Testing

Of all the medical tests for women, pregnancy testing is surely near the top of the most-wanted list. Until recently, women had to leave a urine sample with their doctor, who then forwarded it to a medical laboratory for testing. Now do-it-yourself pregnancy testing kits are available in drugstores for about $10. These offer obvious advantages including privacy and a speedy diagnosis as early as the ninth day after the day you expected your period to begin. All of them check for the presence of a special pregnancy hormone in the urine. When used according to the instructions, they are purportedly 97 percent accurate.

These kits typically consist of a test tube containing special reagent chemicals, a vial of purified water, a dropper with a squeeze bulb, and a test-tube holder. The test is relatively simple to perform and involves placing a few drops of a first-morning urine sample in the test tube, adding the purified water, and shaking vigorously. Then you place the test tube in its special holder, let it stand undisturbed for two hours, and then read the results. A dark brown, doughnut-shaped ring in the test-tube solution indicates a positive test for pregnancy.

If you test positive you should see a doctor, because early prenatal care is essential for both you and the developing baby. All major cities and most small ones have agencies and clinics that provide gynecological advice and services if you can't afford your own doctor. In the event of unwanted, unprotected sex, there is a morning-after treatment that can be effective in avoiding pregnancy if administered within twelve hours of the event. Go to a hospital emergency room if you can't see your own doctor at once.

Breast Self-Examination

One of the most widely recognized tests for detecting cancer in women is self-examination of the breasts. This involves a monthly examination in which you observe and feel for characteristic changes in the breast that indicate the presence of a growth that was not there before.

Many women mistakenly assume that a test they can do themselves is probably inferior to a doctor's examination. Actually, quite the opposite is true in this case. If you examine your breasts thoroughly and faithfully each month, you are in a much better posi-

tion to detect small changes than your doctor who only does an examination once a year. In fact, many more breast cancers are discovered by women themselves than by any physician or sophisticated breast-cancer detection method. If the cancer is caught early, the chances are excellent you can be completely cured of the disease. The key element is time—the longer a cancer has to grow and spread to other parts of the body, the harder it is to cure. Thus any suspicious changes you may discover in your monthly examination should be treated as a medical emergency. While most lumps in the breast turn out to be benign—that is, noncancerous—a lump should always be assumed suspicious until proved otherwise by your doctor.

A word or two here about the anatomy of the breast may help you to better understand what you will see and feel in your self-examination. The breasts contain a substantial amount of fat. Large breasts contain more fat than smaller breasts. This fat is interspersed with fine, ligamentous structures that give the breast its shape and prevent it from sagging. In older women, this ligamentous structure becomes somewhat stretched so that the breasts have a tendency to sag a bit. The breasts also contain alveolar glands, each with its own duct called a lactiferous duct. The glands produce milk when a baby is born, and the ducts transport the milk to the surface in the center of the nipple area.

In the nonlactating breast—that is, a breast that is not producing milk—the milk glands are small, pea-sized structures distributed more or less randomly around the central area of the breast. You may be able to feel some of them. Because the milk

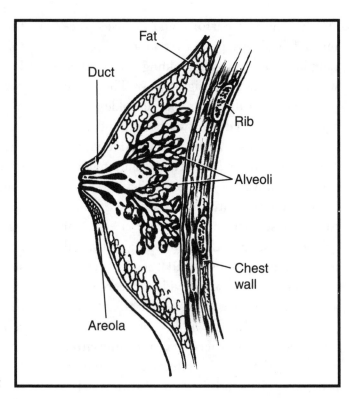

Structures of the Breast

glands are buried in the fat structure, you will not feel them on the surface of the breast tissue but, rather, deep inside. They are not particularly tender to the touch and their size does not vary significantly from month to month.

It is easy at first to mistake the milk glands for tumors, and it is a fact that most breast tumors do grow either in the milk glands themselves or in the duct structures. But as you become familiar with your own breasts, you will know which milk glands can be felt; consequently, you will be able to recognize an abnormal lump that wasn't there before.

All women should examine their breasts on a regular monthly basis. This is best performed about one week after the end of the menstrual period. At this time, the breasts are usually neither tender nor swollen. The swelling and tenderness of the breasts that often accompany the menstrual period are caused by cyclic hormonal changes. After menopause, these changes no longer occur and breast self-examination should be carried out on a regular calendar basis, such as on the first of each month. If a woman is no longer having menstrual periods because of a hysterectomy, she should check with her doctor about the best time to perform breast self-examination. If she is still relatively young and the hysterectomy did not involve both ovaries, her body will still be undergoing cyclic hormonal changes and the breasts should not be examined during the swollen, tender period. If both ovaries have been removed, she will likely be receiving some kind of hormone therapy and instructions about breast self-examination should be sought from the doctor.

A complete breast self-exam consists of three parts that are described in the following sections: an examination by feel while standing, observation in front of a mirror, and examination by feel while lying down.

Examining Your Breasts by Feeling While Standing

1. Breast self-examination should be performed with the hand flat and the fingers together. Do not approach the examination timidly with the tips of one or two fingers or by pinching bits of tissue between the thumb and forefinger. The examination will be much more successful if all four fingers, flattened together, are used.

2. Do the examination during a shower or bath when your hands can glide easily over the wet, soapy skin. With your fingers flat, move your hand gently over every part of the breast and check for any lumps, hard knots, or thickening. Use the right hand to examine the left breast and the left hand to examine the right breast. Do not limit your examination to just the central part of the breast. Cover the entire area from the middle of your chest to the middle of the side of your body, including the armpits. Also be sure you examine both high enough and low enough.

3. Get to know your breasts. If in the first examination you discover one or two particular milk glands, try to identify them again another day. It is very unlikely that you will find a tumor on the first examination; the success of the technique depends on each woman learning the normal anatomy of her own breasts and then perhaps some day discovering that there has been a change in the normal anatomy and that something new has appeared.

Examining Your Breasts by Observing

1. Stand in front of a mirror and inspect your breasts with your arms at your sides. Both breasts will not appear to be the same. One will probably hang a little lower than the other, and one may be a trifle larger than the other. Few women have breasts that, on careful examination, are identical. Observe the contour of your breasts. Look for any swelling, lumps, dimpling of the skin, or any changes in the nipples. These are all important.

2. After observing your breasts with your arms at your sides, raise your arms straight up over your head and hold them high. This lifts up the breasts and changes their shape a bit. Again, look at the shape and contour of each breast for indications of swelling, dimpling of the skin, or changes in the nipple. You may see some changes with your arms held

high over your head that are not apparent when your arms are at your sides.

3. Next, rest the palms of your hands on your hips and press down firmly. This tightens your chest muscles and further modifies the contour and shape of the breasts. Again, look for swelling, lumps, dimpling of the skin, and changes in the nipple. Skin changes and dimpling of the skin are just as significant as lumps. As explained earlier, the breasts contain many small, ligamentous structures, and a small tumor growing along one of the milk ducts may slightly displace one of these ligaments. The small amount of tension placed on the ligament by the tumor will show itself on the surface as a dimple, even though the tumor itself is not large enough to show on the surface as a lump or swelling. Dimpling and skin changes are, therefore, very important findings.

Any change in the nipple is important for the same reason. The nipple normally sticks out. A small tumor, however, may press on one or two of the milk ducts in such a way that the milk ducts pull the nipple in toward the breast. Thus, if a nipple becomes abnormally inverted, this is probably significant.

Examining Your Breasts While Lying Down

1. Lie down on your bed comfortably on your back. Once again you will be examining your right breast with your left hand and your left breast with your right hand.

Start with the right breast. Place a pillow or fold a towel under your right shoulder and put your right hand behind your head. This position tends to make the breast spread out a bit and distributes the breast tissue more evenly over the chest wall.

2. With the fingers of the left hand held flat, press gently around the breast in clockwise motion. Starting at the top of your breast where twelve o'clock might be on a clock face, move around the clock until you have made a full circle back to twelve. A ridge of firm tissue in the lower curve is perfectly normal. Be sure you follow the outer edge of the breast far enough out toward the armpit.

3. When you have made the first complete circle, move about one inch in toward the nipple and start another circle at twelve o'clock. Continue making concentric circles until you have examined every part of your breast including the nipple. This generally requires four or five circles. Because you are looking for relatively small lumps, be sure not to make the space between the circles too large. Also, do not ignore the nipples. Breast tumors can occur in any area of the breast, including directly under the nipple structure.

4. When you have finished examining the right breast, place the towel or pillow under your left shoulder, put your left

hand behind your head, and examine your left breast with your right hand, repeating the procedure described previously.

In this step of the examination you will be looking mostly for lumps. You will always find plenty of lumps that are the normal gland tissue within the breast. After a few examinations you will learn to recognize these gland structures and you will begin to know the location of many of the glands in both your breasts. Some women's breasts are normally much lumpier than others, so don't be alarmed if you find a great many lumps in your breasts and a friend reports finding very few in hers.

5. Finally, squeeze each nipple gently between the thumb and index finger. Normally, nothing should come out. Any discharge, either clear or bloody, should be reported to your doctor.

Once you have been examining your breasts on a regular basis, any abnormality that you find is most likely to start out as something quite small and this is when you want to discover it. Don't expect a lump the size of a golf ball or even a cherry to suddenly show up. You are much more likely to find something the size of an orange seed or smaller that you haven't noticed before. Pay attention to the consistency of the little lumps that are your normal milk glands. If you find something suspicious, it is likely to have a consistency somewhat different, often harder, than that of your normal gland structures. However, consistency is not an infallible indi-

cator of a tumor and you should be much more concerned with finding a small lump in a location where you are quite certain no lumps existed the previous month. Remember, you are primarily looking for changes.

Male Reproductive Organs

Unlike the female, who must go to some lengths just to view the outer fringes of her reproductive system, the male can easily examine his primary sexual organs—the penis and the two testicles contained in the scrotum. The path of the sperm from the testicles to the penis, however, is by no means as direct as many men imagine. Along the way are a number of related organs and glands located within the body cavity and connected by a considerable amount of plumbing in the form of ducts and tubes.

The sperm that ultimately fertilize the female egg are manufactured in the two testicles. These are contained in a small sac called the scrotum, which hangs outside the main body cavity, just behind and below the penis. This arrangement provides precise temperature control for the production of healthy sperm by allowing the testicles to draw close to the body for warmth or drop down to cool off. From the tubules where they are manufactured, the sperm move into the epididymis, a sort of holding area within the scrotum that curves over the back and top of each testicle. Here the immature sperm can mature before continuing on to the vasa deferentia (singular: vas deferens).

The vasa deferentia are the two ducts that conduct the sperm out of the testicles and up into the main body cavity. These

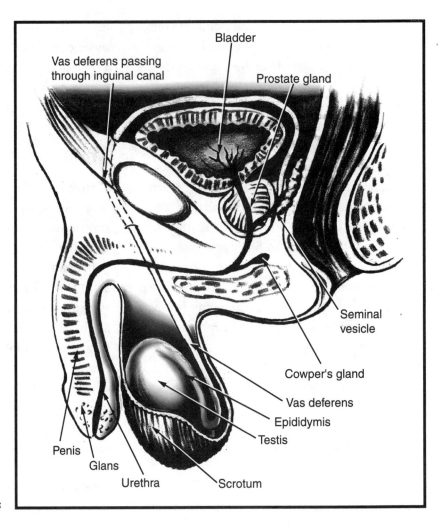

Male Reproductive Organs

slender ducts circle around the bladder, enlarge just a bit to form the ampulla, and then narrow into the ejaculatory ducts that pierce the back of the prostate. The prostate is a gland about the size of a walnut that is situated at the neck of the bladder and surrounds the urethra, through which urine passes. Directly below the ampulla, which is the expanded portion of the vas deferens, is a pouchlike structure called the seminal vesicle. This gland makes and secretes fluid that feeds into the ejaculatory duct, where it

mixes with sperm from the ampullar portion of the vas.

Up to this point, the male reproductive organs have been paired—two testicles, two epididymides, two vasa deferentia, two ampullae, two seminal vesicles, two ejaculatory ducts. But at the site of the prostate everything leaves through one tube—the urethra. The urethra exits to the outside through the penis, which is an erectile organ composed chiefly of spongelike tissue. When sexually aroused, this spongelike tissue becomes engorged with blood, causing the penis to become firm and erect. During ejaculation, the ejaculatory ducts empty into the urethra, the prostate gland contributes some fluids of its own, and the mixture, called semen, is forced out the urethra by muscular contractions. At the same time, a circular muscle around the neck of the bladder closes tightly to prevent urine from passing into the urethra or semen from backing up into the bladder.

To many men the whole process is nothing short of miraculous, and the fear that something might threaten its continued functioning is never far from their minds. Usually, such fears are greatly exaggerated. But it's a good idea nevertheless to keep a weather eye on this vital area by periodically performing the following tests, checks, and examinations.

Checking the Scrotum, Testicles, and the Inguinal Crease

A good place to begin is the scrotum. First, check to see that both testicles have descended into the scrotal sac; it is not uncommon for young boys, or adults for that matter, to have an undescended testicle. This condition should be seen by a doctor.

Compare the relative size of the two testicles—they should be approximately equal, each being about the size of a small plum. The left testicle normally hangs a bit lower than the right. Gently palpate both testicles and note if there is any extreme sensitivity. Now examine the entire scrotum for lumps. Virtually any kind of a lump or mass that appears within the scrotum is abnormal.

Small, relatively hard lumps that suddenly appear within the scrotum may be the first sign of a malignant tumor and medical attention should be sought immediately. Small lumps that appear in the inguinal area—that is, in the crease where the legs join the body—are likely to be swollen lymph nodes. These nodes can swell for a variety of reasons that often have nothing to do with the genitals. For example, an infection in a leg or foot can cause swelling of the lymph nodes in the inguinal area on that side of the body. If these lumps persist, they should be shown to a doctor.

Inguinal Hernia

A soft mass within or just above the scrotum may be due to an inguinal hernia. A hernia is a portion of tissue or part of an organ that has protruded through a weakness or abnormal opening in any part of the body. One of the most common hernias, called an inguinal hernia, involves a loop of bowel that has worked its way into the inguinal canal. This is also discussed in Chapter 3 on the digestive system.

Up until a month or so before birth, the testicles of the male fetus are situated in the abdomen. The inguinal canals are the natural passages through which they descend into the scrotum. This happens shortly before or shortly after birth, after which the passages close. Occasionally, however, the inguinal canals do not close completely and remain as weak spots in the abdominal wall. Any strain causing increased abdominal pressure—such as heavy lifting, violent games, chronic cough, or constipation—can accentuate this weakness and eventually reopen a canal. As continued pressure increases the size of the opening, a loop of bowel can work its way into the passage and eventually enter the scrotum. While this condition can take many years of straining and pushing to develop, inguinal hernias are as common in boys as in grown men.

A hernia is a serious finding because of the possibility that the loop of bowel may become twisted, cutting off the supply of blood to that portion of tissue. This is called a strangulated hernia and necessitates emergency surgery.

Testing for Hernia

A soft mass in the scrotum or in the area just above either testicle may be an inguinal hernia. One test you can do that indicates a hernia condition is to try to "reduce" the mass by manipulating the loop of bowel so that it slides back up into the abdominal cavity.

Lie down on your back with your feet elevated and gently manipulate the mass with your fingers. Generally, an inguinal hernia can be maneuvered back into the abdomen. If this is not possible, the mass may be a hydrocele (see the following section) instead of a hernia.

A second test you can do to check for hernia is the cough test. Stand in front of a full-length mirror, naked, so that you have a good view of the genital area. Now, cough hard and strain in the abdominal area. As you do this, watch the groin area just above the scrotum for a bulge that was not apparent before, or ask someone to watch closely

for you. Any bulge in the area of the groin that is induced by coughing should be checked by your doctor.

A Test for a Hydrocele

A soft mass in the scrotum may also indicate a hydrocele. A hydrocele is a cystic accumulation of fluid within a little sac that forms above the testicle in the scrotum. While this is not a dangerous condition, it can cause considerable discomfort and should be brought to the attention of your physician.

You can test to determine if a mass in the scrotum is a hydrocele using an ordinary flashlight. Switch the flashlight on and press it up tight against the back side of the scrotum. If the mass lights up and glows like a dull, red-orange lightbulb, it is most likely a hydrocele. If, however, light is not transmitted through the mass, it is more likely to be a hernia or some other growth.

Testing for a Varicocele

Each of the testicles in the scrotum is suspended by a cordlike structure consisting of the vas deferens, through which sperm pass, and a number of veins, arteries, lymphatic vessels, and nerves. This structure is called the spermatic cord and the veins that contribute to it are referred to as the testicular veins. These testicular veins can become varicose—that is, enlarged and dilated. This condition is known as a varicocele and occurs almost exclusively in the left spermatic cord.

The presence of a varicocele is indicated by a swelling in the upper scrotum coupled with an abnormal tenderness of the spermatic cord on that side. To check for this condition, locate the spermatic cords on each side of the scrotum. You can easily feel this structure about midway between the testicle and the point at which the scrotum joins the body. Gently palpate the cord between your thumb and forefinger. A light touch here should not cause undue discomfort. If, however, you perceive a noticeable swelling that is painful to the touch, you should have your physician examine the cord for a possible varicocele.

Recognizing Prostate Trouble

The prostate gland contributes some important nutrients to the seminal fluid that provide nourishment for the sperm as they swim up the female vaginal tract toward the egg. Its design, however, is generally counted as one of nature's engineering nightmares. The prostate is located at the base of the bladder, where it surrounds the urethra like a doughnut. When this gland enlarges, as it frequently does, it can effectively slow and eventually shut off the flow of urine from the bladder. If left untreated, severe discomfort and eventual damage to the bladder and kidneys can result.

It has been estimated that at least 50 percent of all men over the age of fifty are likely to develop some form of prostate trouble, and the risk accelerates with advancing age. Prostate disorders fall into three categories:

Infectious prostatitis is an inflammation of the prostate gland caused by a bacterial or a viral infection; the *Escherichia coli* bacilli found in the lower bowel and feces and the gonococcus bacilli are two common offenders here. Benign prostatic hypertrophy, or simply BPH, is an enlargement of the prostate gland that is not cancerous. Prostate cancer, a malignant enlargement of the prostate, is a much rarer condition than simple hypertrophy.

Because of its location within the body, you cannot perform an effective self-examination of the prostate. A doctor will check the prostate by inserting a gloved finger into the rectum and palpating the gland through the rectal wall to feel for lumps, swellings, or tenderness. Even if you could duplicate this procedure, it is unlikely that you would have sufficient expertise to interpret what you feel. There are, however, some signs and symptoms you can observe that indicate prostate trouble. Some of the more common are:

- Frequent, urgent, and painful or difficult urination that may cause you to get up to go to the bathroom two, three, or more times a night
- Difficulty in beginning to urinate
- A feeling that the bladder has not been emptied completely
- Blood in the urine
- A burning sensation in the urethra upon urination or after ejaculation
- Pain in the lower back or the perineal area (the area between the anus and the scrotum)

Some of these symptoms, of course, can be caused by problems other than disorders of the prostate, such as bladder infections. In any case, you should report such warning signs promptly and accurately to your doctor for a professional evaluation.

The PSA Test and Prostate Cancer

Prostate cancer is still on the rise. It is one of the most common cancers in men. The PSA (prostate specific antigen) test is an extremely important test for problems in the prostate, but it is not what is called a cancer test. The presence of prostate specific antigens in your blood will go up with an inflammatory condition in the prostate just as much as it will go up with cancer. So an elevated PSA does not mean you have prostate cancer; it means that something is wrong with the prostate that needs further investigation. It might be cancer or some form of prostatitis.

Prostatitis is treated with antibiotics while prostate cancer is treated with surgery, radiation, or a number of other options that are worked out in careful discussions with you, your primary-care physician, a urologist, and perhaps an oncologist (cancer specialist).

PSA testing has another "if" attached to it. While a positive result may not be caused by cancer, a negative result may not completely free you from the possibility of cancer. A small cancer that is still encapsulated within the prostate may not elevate the PSA reading. But a cancerous (or benign) growth within the prostate can still be felt by the direct rectal exam with a gloved and lubricated finger as described previously. If such a growth or swelling is found, it must be biopsied to determine if it is cancer or something benign such as a calcification. A biopsy, of course, is the removal of a tissue sample from the prostate that is then examined microscopically.

The point is that both PSA testing and a digital rectal exam are musts for men in the forty-five to fifty age range and beyond. Generally, prostate cancer is much more aggressive when it appears in younger men. The older you are when it is discovered, the less chance there is for rapid spreading. That's why in older men the doctor will try to determine whether you are likely to die of something else long before a prostate cancer will get you and will design a treatment accordingly.

Sexually Transmitted Diseases in Men

Genital Warts

As in the female, genital warts in the male thrive on moisture. Thus penile discharges, sweat, and other secretions provide the warts with an environment that must seem made-to-order. Look for small clusters of pinkish-tan growths not much larger than grains of rice on the penis, the scrotum, and around the anus. They begin small, but they can dramatically mushroom into large, cauliflowerlike masses. Scratching can spread the infection and sexual intercourse can pass it on to your partner.

Genital Herpes

This also follows a similar course in men and women. The first sign is likely to be several small, red bumps on the penis that generally appear two to eight days after intercourse with an infected person. These bumps quickly escalate into tiny, painful blisters filled with a clear fluid. As white blood cells move into the blisters to combat the virus, this fluid becomes cloudy. At this stage the blisters rupture, leaving small, wet open sores that are still painful and still infectious. About ten days after their first appearance, the sores crust over, pain gradually subsides, and healing follows. The entire episode is often accompanied by fever, swollen lymph glands in the groin, and burning on urination. A relapse may strike about six to eight weeks later, and subsequent episodes can recur periodically throughout life, though these are usually less severe than the initial bout.

Syphilis

Detecting primary syphilis in men, as in women, involves finding its characteristic sore, called a chancre, on the genitals, mouth, or anus. The chancre is painless, round, and slightly raised and has a hard base that may feel as if there is a coin embedded in the skin. It lasts about two to six weeks and then heals by itself, even without treatment. Long before this, however, the spirochete that causes syphilis has entered the bloodstream.

Syphilis may be detected during its secondary stage by a generalized skin rash that appears anywhere from a few days to a few weeks after the chancre heals. Either of these symptoms or merely the suspicion that you have been exposed to syphilis should prompt a visit to your doctor for a confirmed diagnosis and treatment. (A more detailed description of the rash of secondary syphilis is included in Chapter 9, which deals with skin problems.) The next stage of syphilis involves invasion of other body organs with extremely serious consequences.

Gonorrhea

While gonorrhea in women often goes unnoticed at first, a gonorrheal infection in men usually announces its presence within a week after exposure with two unmistakable symptoms that often encourage a man to go to the doctor. The first is a discharge of pus from the opening of the penis, and the second is a burning sensation when passing urine. Other infections, some sexually acquired and some not, can cause the same symptoms. In any case, they should be seen by a doctor.

As mentioned earlier, simple culture tests for gonorrhea exist and may one day join other self-diagnosis kits, such as pregnancy and urine testing, on drugstore shelves. Left untreated or self-treated with folk or street remedies, gonorrhea can cause sterility and other nasty problems.

HIV and AIDS

Infection with the human immunodeficiency virus (HIV) and the acquired immunodeficiency syndrome (AIDS) that results from it are more strictly classified as general infectious diseases rather than sexually transmitted diseases, but they appear here because sexual contact with an infected person accounts for a large proportion of the transmission of the virus. The virus is also transmitted by intravenous drug users who share needles and by an infected pregnant mother to her fetus. A very small percentage of cases (perhaps 0.5 percent) are transmitted in other ways—usually by some form of contact with blood from an infected person. No HIV transmission or AIDS cases have been traced to casual contact, coughing, sneezing, or touching.

Viruses are more intractable when it comes to finding treatment for them because antibiotic drugs have no effect. Thus, when you go to the doctor coughing, sneezing, and complaining of a bad cold, he or she will not treat you with antibiotics if it is determined you have a viral infection, but you will be treated with antibiotics if you have a bacterial infection—pneumonia or strep throat, for example. Eradication of viral diseases has always come from finding vaccines that prevent infections rather than from drugs that cure. Smallpox, polio, and measles are examples of viruses that have been successfully controlled with vaccines. The human immunodeficiency virus is particularly elusive because it seems to contin-

ually change its structure and can invade healthy cells without the body's immune defenses being aware of it.

This is not to say that nothing can be done. When HIV is diagnosed before it has developed into AIDS, aggressive treatment can delay the onset of the disease for years and can help a person fight off diseases that are secondary to AIDS—that is, that are caused by the virus's attack on the immune system. And with the vigorous attention being given to finding a vaccine against HIV and curative agents for AIDS, hopefully the information you are now reading will be history within a few years.

Anyone who suspects he or she has been exposed to HIV should be tested. Confidential testing is available through many community medical facilities and there is also a test you can buy in the drugstore for about $30. This test involves applying blood from a finger prick to chemically treated paper. You send the paper that is identified only with a number to a laboratory in a preaddressed envelope. After about a week you call the laboratory for the results. It is a totally confidential procedure. In the event of a positive result, you should go to your physician or a health-care agency to verify the diagnosis and begin treatment if necessary. You can find an AIDS hot-line number in the community-services section in the front of your telephone book.

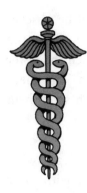

11

Your Endocrine Glands and Metabolism

Endocrine glands are sometimes referred to as glands of internal secretion because the products of these glands are used inside the body to control various metabolic processes. Metabolism is a broad term that refers to the way certain cells in various organs absorb nutrients and produce energy that results in the way the body grows, functions, and repairs itself.

The endocrine system is a series of glands that are controlled by the pituitary gland, which is often referred to as the master gland because of its effects on all the others. The pituitary, a pea-sized gland in the head nestled under the brain, secretes a wide variety of substances that control the secretions of the other glands: the thyroid, the adrenals, the gonads (ovaries and testes), and islet cells in the pancreas, which produce insulin.

Many problems caused by the endocrine glands do not lend themselves to home testing. If there is something wrong with your metabolism, you will probably go to the doctor complaining of a variety of vague symptoms—weight loss or gain, fatigue, hyperactivity, loss of libido, menstrual problems, growth abnormalities in children, and so on—and it often takes a good bit of detective work and laboratory testing to pinpoint the problem. Sometimes many avenues are pursued by the doctor before an endocrine gland is implicated in the problem. Other problems, however, provide clues that you can spot yourself.

The Thyroid Gland

The thyroid gland is a butterfly-shaped gland situated over the trachea, or windpipe, with one "wing" on either side. Its main function is to control metabolism. It does this by producing tiny amounts of hormones that are released into the bloodstream on instructions from the pituitary.

Except in very thin people, it is difficult to actually feel a normal thyroid gland. It is, however, the only gland in the neck that moves when you swallow. Thus, if you locate your Adam's apple and press your fingers lightly but firmly over the area immediately below, you may be able to feel the thyroid gland move beneath your fingers as you drink a glass of water.

The thyroid gland may become enlarged, in which case it is known as a goiter. Men may first notice the presence of a goiter when they have difficulty buttoning a shirt collar. Women may first notice it as a puffiness in the front of the neck. Such a swelling may feel hard or soft, smooth or lumpy, and may vary in size from barely visible to greatly distended. Any thyroid gland that you can locate with your eyes alone, without the aid of the swallow test, is abnormally enlarged and should be examined by your doctor.

The thyroid gland may become either underactive or overactive in its hormone production, and this can happen without any telltale changes in size. A thyroid hormone deficiency, called hypothyroidism, is indicated by a combination of symptoms. These include an increase in the amount of sleep you require every day, a moderate weight gain that is not associated with increased hunger or even increased food intake, dry skin, brittle, coarse hair, and a chronic tired and sluggish feeling. If this picture seems to fit you, the following test is useful in helping to decide if your problem is caused by a thyroid hormone deficiency.

Testing for an Underactive Thyroid

This test involves the knee-jerk reflex that is also described in Chapter 6 on the nervous system. Here, however, you will be observing not so much the knee jerk itself as the relaxation stage of the reflex when the lower leg returns to its normal position. The knee-jerk test is best carried out with some help from an assistant.

1. Sit on a table so that your legs swing freely from the knee joint, with your knees bared.

2. Locate your kneecap with your fingers. This is the rounded bone that sits right over the knee.

3. Next, locate a bony prominence an inch or so below the kneecap. This is the top end of the large bone in your lower leg. In the very front part of your leg you will feel a fairly stiff cord running in this short space between the bottom of the kneecap and the top of the leg bone. You should actually be able to put your thumb and index finger on either side of this cord. You are now holding the tendon you are about to test. Mark this point with an *x* using a felt-tip pen.

4. With your legs totally relaxed, ask your assistant to briskly tap each knee with a rubber reflex hammer at the point you have marked. It is very important to relax or the test will not work properly. Remember, it is a *tap*, not a blow. You can use the handle of a screwdriver for tapping in place of a rubber reflex hammer.

5. In most people, if the test is performed correctly the lower leg will immediately

give a little jerk. Normally, the lower leg will relax promptly. When thyroid hormone production is deficient, however, the leg sinks slowly back to its former position. This sluggish relaxation phase of the deep-tendon reflex is characteristic of an underactive thyroid.

The thyroid gland requires a certain amount of iodine to make the hormone thyroxine, so a goiter can be caused by an iodine deficiency in the diet. With an iodine deficiency the gland works extra hard and enlarges. Goiters used to be rather common, especially in areas far from the ocean where people didn't have access to seafood with its high iodine content. But now that iodine is added to salt and seafood is available everywhere, thanks to modern refrigeration, goiters have become rather uncommon.

The thyroid can become overactive as well as underactive in its production of the hormone governing our metabolism. An overactive thyroid condition is called *hyperthyroidism* and it, too, is characterized by a combination of symptoms.

People suffering from hyperthyroidism almost always lose weight even when they increase their food intake; their skin feels moist, they perspire excessively, their heart rate is rapid, they feel nervous and jittery, and they often exhibit exophthalmia. In common terms, this is called "pop eyes" and it actually looks as if the eyes are slowly bulging out of their sockets. The first sign of this is just a slightly wide-eyed look. Normally the upper eyelid rests over part of the iris, which is the colored part of the eye. But as the eye bulges out, the lid is raised higher and higher and more and more of the upper part of the iris is exposed.

Testing for an Overactive Thyroid

1. Hold one hand out in front of you with the back side up and stretch all the fingers out as far as they will go.

2. Now lay an ordinary sheet of paper on the back of your hand. Watch the edges of this paper carefully. In a few people the edges will remain absolutely still. In most, the edges will wiggle a little. If you have an overactive thyroid, however, the edges of the paper will vibrate quite violently. No matter how still you try to hold your hand, the paper will still dance around.

3. While people may develop hand tremors for many reasons, a significant tremor in combination with a loss of weight, slightly bulging eyes, and a feeling of nervousness suggests hyperthyroidism, and a physician should be consulted.

Hypothyroidism (less than enough thyroxine being produced) is usually treated with hormone-replacement therapy. Because some of the symptoms of hypothyroidism resemble psychiatric depression (especially the tired, lethargic feeling), the thyroid should be checked whenever depression is suspected.

Hyperthyroidism (too much thyroxine being produced) is treated with one of several therapies: medication, radioactive iodine, or surgery to remove part of the thyroid gland.

The Adrenal Glands

There are two adrenal glands, small structures located on the top end of each kidney. The adrenals secrete a number of steroid hormones that affect a variety of body functions: sodium and potassium levels in cells; carbohydrate, fat, and protein metabolism; reaction to stress (adrenaline); and certain influences over the sex organs. A loss of these steroid hormones through adrenal insufficiency can result in general weakness, deficient neuromuscular function, poor resistance to stress, and diminished resistance to infections.

Adrenal insufficiency is known as Addison's disease; weakness and fatigability are among its earliest symptoms. As the disease progresses, the affected person may become somewhat more pigmented—darker in color, that is, especially over the elbows, knees, and knuckles. A number of other symptoms may occur that resemble other ailments, so it may take some detective work for a doctor to diagnose adrenal insufficiency. Fortunately, it is a relatively uncommon condition. Treatment is with hormone replacement or other procedures if tumors on the glands are suspected.

Overactivity of the adrenal glands leads to what is called Cushing's syndrome. The clinical features of Cushing's syndrome are quite characteristic: weight gain, accumulation of fat on the trunk, an enlargement of cheeks and face (moonface), and a swelling on the back of the neck and upper back, often called a buffalo hump. Cushing's syndrome can be caused either by the adrenal glands making too much of their steroid hormones or by the overuse of cortisone-type medicines. It is important to strictly limit the use of prescribed cortisone-type medicines to the exact dosage and length of time ordered by the doctor.

Athletes who take androgenic steroids to supplement what is normally produced by their adrenal glands, in an attempt to improve their performance, are clearly endangering their health.

Insulin and Diabetes

The hormone insulin is produced in a special part of the pancreas called islet cells, whose function is quite distinct from the other function of the pancreas, which is to produce digestive enzymes. Once the pancreas loses its ability to produce insulin, diabetes develops and the affected person will have to take insulin for life, an oral medication, or some combination of the two. Diabetes is by far the most common of the endocrine diseases and is divided into two types, designated as Type I and Type II. Type I is insulin-dependent and the onset of the disease can be at any age. Type II is noninsulin-dependent and most often appears in adult life. It is a condition in which the pancreas continues to produce insulin, but not enough to handle the glucose that the body is creating.

Insulin replacement has to be carefully regulated to match a person's carbohydrate intake. Too little will allow a person's blood sugar to go very high, to the point of becoming ill and lapsing into unconsciousness. Too much insulin, on the other hand, may make the blood-sugar level go so low that, again, the affected person is in danger of losing consciousness. In Type I diabetes, low blood sugar is treated by adding glucose to the body, either by mouth or by intravenous injection, while high blood sugar is treated with insulin.

Control of diet is important in affected people in the management of both Type I and Type II diabetes, and both must check their blood-sugar levels regularly, although the Type II patient may just take medication once or twice a day. New medications are on the horizon for noninsulin-dependent diabetics, and these people should keep themselves informed by reading the literature and discussing their progress with their doctors.

Because of the prevalence of diabetes, one of the most widely used home medical tests is the blood-sugar test kit. A wide variety of these tests is available at any drugstore, and your doctor may want to recommend one that seems best for you. Based on the blood-sugar level indicated by the testing instrument, the diabetic gives him- or herself an appropriate amount of insulin. This is done by self-injection or with an insulin pump. These testing instruments have allowed diabetics to control their blood sugar to nearly normal levels at most times—even when eating junk food at a ball game or dining out in a restaurant.

Testing instruments are small enough to fit in the palm of your hand, which is why they are so convenient to use when eating away from home. They cost between $50 and $100, but they are well worth the investment in the returns they provide by allowing you to control the disease more precisely.

Here are some frightening facts about diabetes—good reason to be aware of whether you have the disease or not and to control it carefully if you do have it:

- More than a half million people are diagnosed with diabetes every year.

- Diabetes is far more common today than it was thirty years ago.

- Type II diabetes is most likely to develop in people over forty who are obese and sedentary and have a family history of the disease.

- Diabetes affects 14 million people in the United States; as many as half of these don't know they have it.

- Diabetes is a leading cause of blindness, stroke, heart disease, kidney disease, and loss of feet and legs to deterioration and subsequent amputation.

One of the typical symptoms of diabetes is excessive and continual thirst and resulting excessive urination. This is not the normal thirst associated with eating spicy foods or doing hot, dusty work nor the urination associated with a night of partying. A diabetic may also experience excessive hunger, weight loss, weakness, and lethargy. An affected person may also experience unexplained episodes of blurred vision, skin disorders, fungal infections, and impotence. In other words, it is a debilitating illness that can affect many organs and body systems.

The Gonads

A number of hormones are produced in the ovaries of a woman and in the testicles of a man, the main ones being estrogen in the female and testosterone in the male.

Production of these hormones is affected by other hormones produced at other sites, resulting in a rather complex series of events that affect sexual characteristics, reproductive functions, and other body operations in ways that are not always fully understood. In cases of sexual dysfunction and infertility, the levels of sex hormones being produced are almost always checked. And at the present time the role that estrogen and testosterone play in diseases associated with aging are the subject of intense investigation and controversy in medical research.

In fact, much of the operation of the entire array of endocrine glands and their effects on each other and on all the organs of the body remain quite mysterious. So when things go chronically wrong with your health that can't be explained in other ways, the functioning of the endocrine system is often a good place to look. Specialists who investigate endocrine functioning are endocrinologists, gynecologists for women experiencing problems with their reproductive organs, and urologists for men experiencing problems with theirs.

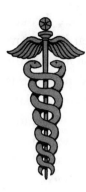

12

A Personal Health-Hazard Appraisal and the Leading Causes of Death

When an insurance company insures your life or your health, it is playing a game of chance with you in a very real sense. The insurance company bets that you are going to stay alive and healthy long enough for it to make a profit from your insurance premiums, while you bet that you are going to get sick or die and collect at least as much money from the insurance company as you have paid in premiums. But just like all professional gamblers, the insurance companies are very adept at appraising the odds.

By looking at your health history and inquiring about your lifestyle, an insurance company actuary can tell you what your prospects are for surviving the next ten years. He or she can say with a pretty fair degree of statistical accuracy whether you are physiologically older or younger than your actual age on your last birthday—that is, what your chances are for living a longer or shorter life than other people your age. Your doctor can do this, too, and so can you.

While your doctor or insurance company can't guarantee life or death for any one individual, your *chances* for survival as compared with others in your population group can be assessed. It is also true that if you are at high risk, especially from those health hazards that account for most of the deaths in your age group, there are things you can do to improve your prospects for living a longer, healthier life.

This is the basis for "preventive medicine" that is so important to insurance companies, to the managed-health-care industry, to government agencies that pay a large part of the national health-care bills, and to your health and well-being. The reason that all these entities undertake massive health-education campaigns is that most aspects of preventive medicine are not the province of doctors but of individuals. While we can't be blamed for health hazards that time and chance expose us to, it is a fact that everyone can have a considerable impact for the better on the fourteen health hazards that account for more than 95 percent of deaths every year (out of some one thousand causes overall). We can have an even greater impact on the enormous social and economic costs created by those left alive but disabled by these health hazards.

The fourteen leading causes of death and disability in the order of the toll they take are: heart disease; cancer; stroke; obstructive lung disease; pneumonia; diabetes; nonautomotive accidents of all types; diseases of the arteries; automobile accidents; suicide; liver disease; homicide; kidney disease; and septicemia (systemic blood poisoning). HIV infections can be added to this list, but the statistics are somewhat indeterminate because HIV-positive people are at risk from many other infectious diseases that may be the ultimate cause of their deaths.

The following table, based on reported deaths from the National Center for Health Statistics (NCHS), shows the fourteen most frequent causes of death for males and females among various age groups. As might be expected, deaths from most diseases increase dramatically with age—heart disease, stroke, and pneumonia are notable among these. But deaths from many causes begin to take a sharp upturn for people in their mid thirties. Accidents, homicides, and suicides rather than diseases are the principal health hazards for teens and young adults, especially among males. Deaths from HIV infections peak among males in their thirties and forties. For most health hazards, men seem to be at greater risk than women; but from age seventy-five up, more women succumb to many of the same health hazards, mostly because more women than men still are alive at this point.

The official NCHS figures are broken down by sex and race. Many hazards are considerably worse for males of color than for others. For example, high blood pressure is a particularly serious threat for young black males. This breakdown is available in most libraries or via the Internet if you would like to see it. We have not included statistical differences by race here because socioeconomic conditions also play an important part in appraising health hazards, and these are much more difficult to take into account. If you are an average individual living in at least moderate circumstances in a relatively stable home environment, the racial statistics will make little difference to you among the general population.

As you will see later in this chapter, while you can't escape every health hazard that fate and perhaps your genes may impose on you, you can play a very important role in helping yourself to avoid or lessen the effects of most of them. On the other hand, your doctor can't prevent any of this; he or she can only advise you how to take care of yourself and then treat you when you are ill.

How to Increase Your Chances for Survival

In a discussion with his heart surgeon at the Mary Hitchcock-Dartmouth Medical Center about who gets heart disease and who doesn't, a patient complained that while he exercised vigorously and was not overweight, he still had needed quintuple bypass surgery, and yet he knew many people who were sedentary, overweight, and ate all the wrong foods and who seemed healthy as young plow horses.

Annual Deaths from Fourteen Leading Causes

	Heart disease	Cancer	Stroke	Obstructive lung disease	Pneumonia	Diabetes	Non-auto accidents	Diseases of the arteries	Auto accidents	Suicide	Liver disease	Homicide	Kidney disease	Septicemia
Male 15–24	771	1,013	94	128	122	66	2,914	40	7,687	4,119	22	7,206	29	30
Female	501	725	114	78	121	52	552	27	2,813	730	17	1,218	19	34
Male 25–34	2,940	2,496	420	136	419	323	4,788	127	6,086	5,218	479	5,686	135	164
Female	1,672	2,583	377	160	297	279	1,022	83	2,126	1,089	242	1,592	85	110
Male 35–44	11,414	7,684	1,365	355	1,000	1,020	5,837	314	4,357	4,842	2,732	3,476	283	357
Female	5,002	9,071	1,154	378	532	677	1,347	216	1,714	1,328	1,024	1,061	175	252
Male 45–54	27,905	21,098	2,742	1,328	1,145	1,917	3,275	682	2,633	3,134	3,451	1,596	441	483
Female	11,371	21,274	2,315	1,166	712	1,532	951	372	1,170	1,034	1,252	456	319	358
Male 55–64	57,453	50,364	5,216	5,771	2,210	3,784	2,470	2,100	1,887	2,372	3,796	734	976	854
Female	28,308	40,321	4,409	4,900	1,448	3,694	1,027	946	1,021	689	1,817	243	878	755
Male 65–74	116,740	91,693	12,966	17,165	6,373	7,013	3,105	5,902	1,756	2,425	3,693	433	2,530	2,071
Female	78,160	71,616	12,345	14,103	4,336	7,971	1,904	3,318	1,360	615	2,401	258	2,250	1,926
Male 75–84	144,632	77,248	21,455	20,982	13,099	6,617	3,744	7,493	1,714	2,003	1,746	183	3,831	2,940
Female	158,468	69,289	29,910	17,318	12,502	9,705	3,731	6,652	1,476	387	1,745	196	3,976	3,549
Male 85+	89,596	26,789	14,592	8,357	12,777	2,671	2,878	4,683	594	646	324	54	2,851	1,820
Female	211,406	34,914	40,283	8,500	23,862	6,525	5,101	10,275	421	132	417	85	4,305	4,540
Male Totals	451,451	278,385	58,850	54,222	37,145	23,411	29,011	21,341	26,714	24,759	16,243	19,368	11,076	8,719
Female	494,888	249,793	90,907	46,603	43,810	30,435	15,635	21,889	12,101	6,004	8,915	5,109	12,007	11,524

"Don't worry," the surgeon said, "I'll get to see most of them—the ones who get here in time, that is."

What this conversation illustrates is that not everyone will succumb to heart disease who does everything contrary to modern medical advice, as the patient correctly observed. Some few will live to a healthy old age without giving a thought to what they eat or what they do—everyone can point to examples of people they know who are like this. But it is also true, as the surgeon observed, that chances are good that he will see many of them for bypass surgery and that many others will die untimely deaths before medical intervention can help. Still others will spend their declining years disabled and dependent because of badly diseased arteries.

The art of medical prognostication is not an exact science—there are more unknowns than knowns at this point in medical history in the way the body works and responds to inside and outside influences—but actuarial statistics are quite good at predicting your chances for good health and long life among others of your age and kind. So you can bet with the odds among the general population or bet on yourself as a long shot. More people who bet with the odds will live longer, healthier lives, but they will have to expend some effort and discipline in the meantime. Those who want to bet they will be among the favored few who will live long and healthy lives without worrying about the annoying details of a healthy lifestyle may indeed be among the winners in the game of survival, but they should be aware that their chances are not good and no one in the health and survival business would be willing to bet on them.

The following health-hazard appraisal can give you some idea of what your risks are for falling heir to the leading causes of death and disability as compared with the rest of the population. After age seventy-four, an age factor kicks in for most of the health risks, but even at this point you can still see how other risk factors may affect your general well-being.

Heart Disease, Diseases of the Arteries, and Stroke

In the decade from age thirty-five to forty-four, heart and artery diseases become the leading health hazards and the number one causes of death, surpassing the primary scourges of youth—accidents, homicide, and suicide. The lifestyle and genetic factors that have been shown to increase the risk of these diseases are too well known by now to need repeating, but you might be interested in seeing how these factors can affect your chances for succumbing to them.

If your total of the risk factors (see next page) is below 8, your risk for heart and artery diseases is lower than the general population; 8 indicates an average risk factor; 9 to 12 suggests you are slightly above the average person's risk; over 12 indicates medical attention and lifestyle changes are needed.

Cancer

The table showing the fourteen leading causes of death lumps all deaths from cancer together although the NCHS keeps track of deaths from more than sixty malignant neoplasms—that is, new masses of cells in

Risk Factors for Heart and Artery Diseases and Stroke

Risk	Risk Factor	Your Risk Factor	Risk	Risk Factor	Your Risk Factor
Systolic Blood Pressure			Exercise		
200 or more	3		Little or none	3	
180	2.5		Regular and		
160	2		moderate	1	
140	1.5		Regular and		
130	1		vigorous	0.5	_____
125 or less	0.5	_____	Parents Who Died of		
Diastolic Blood Pressure			Heart or Artery Disease		
100 or more	3.5		Before Age 65		
90	1.5		Both	2	
Less than 90	1	_____	One	1.5	
Cholesterol Ratio			Neither	1	_____
(Total cholesterol ÷ HDL cholesterol)			Smoking		
5 or above	2.5		Cigarettes	2.5	
4.0–4.5	1		Cigars, pipe, chewing	2	
below 4.0	0.5	_____	No tobacco	1	_____
Diabetes			Weight		
Yes, and poorly			75 percent or more		
looked after	3		overweight	2.5	
Yes, but carefully			50 percent overweight	2	
controlled	2		15 percent overweight	1	
No diabetes	1	_____	Recommended weight	0.5	_____
			Your Total of Risk Factors		_____

the body that show abnormal and uncontrolled growth.

What causes malignant neoplasms has been the subject of the most intense investigation for many decades with no really definitive answers available at this writing. Scientists are zeroing in on certain genetic links that hold promise for providing some answers, and statistical studies seem to leave little doubt that there is a considerably higher risk among smokers for a variety of cancers. Ultraviolet rays have been implicated in skin cancers, and exposure to radioactive materials seems to increase the risks for a variety of cancers.

Because the death rate for a number of cancers has declined as a result of new and better treatments, early detection is vital in increasing your chances for survival. If any of

Risk Factors for Cancer

Risk	Risk Factor	Your Risk Factor	Risk	Risk Factor	Your Risk Factor
Frequent Use of Any Tobacco			You self-test plus regularly complete medical exams that include cancer screenings	1	_____
Heavy use	3				
Moderate use	2				
No use at all	0.5	_____			
			Lifestyle		
Early Warning Tests			You give no consideration to what you eat or drink	3	
You rarely have a regular physical checkup and rarely self-test	3		You have some concern about low-fat, high-fiber eating and limiting alcohol consumption	2	
You self-test only	2.5		You try conscientiously to follow a healthy regimen	1	_____
You have medical checkups but don't include such things as prostate test or Pap smear, mammogram, occult blood in stool, check of rectum and lower bowel	2.5		**Age**		
			Over forty	2	
			Under forty	1	_____

Your Total of Risk Factors　　_____

your risk factors are more than 1, you should want to reappraise how you protect yourself against letting some form of cancer get an undetected start on you.

Chronic Obstructive Lung Diseases

Emphysema is the biggest health hazard in this category, which also includes asthma,

chronic bronchitis, and diseases resulting from prolonged breathing of dust (such as happens to miners, cotton processors, and asbestos workers) and other pollutants.

There is little to appraise here: If you smoke or breathe polluted air on a regular basis, you are at very high risk. If you have asthma and fail to follow your doctor's orders religiously, you are at high risk. If you do two or more of these things, you are at extremely high risk of early disability and death.

Diabetes

The table showing the fourteen leading causes of death lists diabetes as the sixth leading cause of death. This is not the whole picture, however. These are deaths that can be attributed directly to the diabetes— adverse reactions to too much or too little sugar in the blood that have resulted in coma and death. Other statistics point to 160,000 deaths annually where the end cause might be heart attack, stroke, kidney disease, and other complications brought on by the diabetes. In addition, many thousands of diabetics are disabled by resulting blindness, nerve damage, and amputation of limbs.

It is estimated that diabetes is three times as common today as it was forty years ago, and no one is quite sure why. More good food and less exercise would seem to be major culprits as the good times rolled on for four consecutive decades, but this is speculation. Many people whose lifestyles are entirely praiseworthy get Type I or Type II diabetes. Genetic susceptibility probably plays an important role.

The good news is that steady and noteworthy progress is constantly being made in controlling diabetes so that most diabetics can

Risk Factors for Diabetes

Risk	Risk Factor	Your Risk	Risk	Risk Factor	Your Risk
Weight			Doctor has advised blood sugar is normal	1	_____
75% overweight	3				
50% overweight	2.5		Exercise		
25% overweight	2		Little or no exercise	2.5	
10% overweight	1		Moderate regular exercise	1	
Recommended weight or less	0.5	_____	Vigorous regular exercise	0.5	_____
Doctor Involvement			Parents		
Diagnosed diabetic with no control effort made	5		Two parents with diabetes	2	
Diagnosed diabetic with some effort at control	3		One parent with diabetes	1.5	
Diagnosed diabetic with diligent program for control	1.5		No parent with diabetes	1	_____
Don't know blood-sugar level	1.5				
			Your Total of Risk Factors		_____

have as good an outlook for longevity as anyone else if they diligently cooperate with the physicians, therapists, and dieticians who show them how to control the disease. But, of course, before diabetes can be controlled it must be discovered. While there are approximately 14 million diabetics in the United States, only half of them are aware that they have the disease. Some conditions would seem to put people at greater risk for diabetes than others, and these are listed in the chart.

Whatever your total of risk factors is, you should discuss your standing in relation to diabetes with your doctor during your next checkup if you haven't done so before. If your total of risk factors is six or more, you should discuss your standing in relation to diabetes with your doctor without fail, and the subject should be revisited regularly. A score of eight or more indicates you are at considerable risk and that you should work out a program with your doctor for adjusting your lifestyle.

Pneumonia and Liver Diseases

Pneumonia and liver diseases can strike anyone regardless of their lifestyles or how they take care of their health. Certain varieties of hepatitis, for example, may be acquired in some long-forgotten incident in childhood that devastates the liver in later life. And it is not uncommon for an otherwise healthy person to develop pneumonia following an illness.

Lifestyle, however, does play an important role in the risk from these diseases in some obvious circumstances. People who are weakened or run-down are more susceptible to pneumonia than others. Older people and those with debilitating diseases should be wary of influenza and get an annual flu shot. Young people who may be stressed or undernourished can develop pneumonia following a cold more easily than someone who is fit. Lack of caution when traveling in an underdeveloped country can result in a case of hepatitis that affects the liver.

Alcoholics and intravenous drug users are particularly susceptible to liver diseases, accounting for at least a third of deaths from this cause. And the weakened condition these addicts are in also makes them susceptible to pneumonia and a variety of other diseases. Cigarette smokers and people with emphysema are at considerably higher risk for pneumonia than others.

Keeping yourself generally fit, being conscious of how your body systems are operating, and taking any disease-preventive steps your doctor may recommend are really the only ways you can reduce your risks from these diseases.

Accidents

Automobile accidents and all other kinds of accidents share so many of the same risk factors that we have combined them here. It is rather strange that despite some hundred thousand deaths caused by accidents every year, plus uncountable injuries and permanent disabilities suffered, most people don't think of accidents as health hazards.

The major risks for accidents include youth, use of alcohol and other drugs, and a love affair with speed or other reckless behavior. Certain occupations, of course, are riskier than others. Because more men than women work at hazardous occupations, because more men than women enjoy risky pleasures, because more men than women speed on the highway, and because more men than women drink before driving, three to five times as many men die as the result of accidents as women. Deaths from automobile accidents are at their highest from ages sixteen to thirty-five, while deaths from all other accidents are highest from ages twenty-five to fifty-five, the prime working years for men engaged in hazardous occupations.

These, then, are your risks for death from accidents:

A total of five or less puts you at much less risk from death by accident than the rest of your age group. A score of ten indicates you are at high risk of death by accident; more than ten puts you at very high risk and you should review your lifestyle if you want to increase your chances for surviving the next ten years.

Suicide and Homicide

These are two more risks that we don't think of as health hazards even though these violent events take more than 55,000 lives a year. In every age group, men are two to five times as likely to be murdered as

Risk Factors for Accidents

Risk	Risk Factor	Your Risk Factor	Risk	Risk Factor	Your Risk Factor
Age			Occupation		
15 to 25	5		Considered hazardous	5	
26 to 55	3		Moderately hazardous	2	
Over 55	1	_____	Nonhazardous	1	_____
Gender			Attitude		
Male	3		Like to speed on highways	5	
Female	1	_____	Enjoy the rush of risk taking	5	
Alcohol and Drugs			Impatient by nature or easily upset	4	
Sometimes excessive	5		None of the above	1	_____
Always very moderate	1				
Nonuser	0.5	_____			

Your Total of Risk Factors _____

women. The murder rate among black Americans is four times that of the rest of the population. But regardless of race, you are at greater risk of death from murder if you are male and young (under age fifty-five), live in poverty, and have access to a gun. If you have been arrested for a felony or if you carry a gun or a knife, your risk of murder soars in relation to the rest of the population.

Depression and a family history of suicide are the highest risk factors in this category. Untreated mental depression is also a risk factor in other diseases because it seems to impact on the functioning of the immune system and also causes people to neglect themselves. Given the effect that depression and other mental illnesses have on general health, it is hard to understand why health insurers are currently so reluctant to pay for mental-health maintenance and treatment as a preventive for other costly diseases.

Something to think about: Seventy percent of deaths among boys fifteen to nineteen are caused by motor-vehicle accident, suicide, homicide, and other violent events. If any disease were to take this toll on our youth, the country would be in a state of panic greater than that experienced in the polio epidemics of the early twentieth century or the plagues of the Middle Ages.

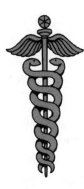

13

How to Create Your Own Medical History

Every medical testing program must begin with a comprehensive medical history, whether a doctor does it or you do it yourself. As you will see, there are many reasons why a well-kept personal record is a valuable health document and is usually superior to a patchwork of professional records scattered around the country among many doctors. It is the means by which you track the performance of your body systems and keep an eye on your health habits—and it plays no small role in keeping you well, in heading off serious illness, and in prolonging your life. In addition, a complete and documented personal health history is the most important diagnostic tool you can give to a doctor when you go to seek treatment.

Not long ago, a study was conducted in England to determine the relative values of a medical history, a physical examination, and laboratory tests in diagnosing a patient's condition. First, doctors at a general medical clinic were asked to diagnose their cases after they had done nothing more than take a careful medical history. They were asked again for the most likely diagnosis after they had conducted a physical examination, and again after they had the results of all the tests and x-rays they had ordered.

In about 85 percent of the cases, the doctors made correct diagnoses on the basis of the medical histories alone! The physical examinations increased the correct diagnosis rate by only 5 percent, and the medical tests by only 5 percent more. Finally, when all the data was available, no certain diagnosis could be made in the remaining 5 percent of patients.

The study concluded that the medical history gives doctors most of the information they need to make correct diagnoses, while examinations and tests serve to make the doctors' opinions more conclusive and supply the confidence needed to prescribe appropriate treatments.

What Is a Medical History?

A medical history may be started from the response to a single question such as "Well, now, what seems to be the trouble?" or it may be a complete record of everything medically significant in your life from the time you were born. It depends on what you and your doctor expect to accomplish together. If you are making a transient visit to the doctor with an injured thumb, or if you are seeking relief from what is obviously a head cold, neither you nor the doctor will want to spend a lot of time on the history of your life. But if your problem seems to be serious or puzzling, if you are seeking a complete appraisal of your health, or if you expect the doctor to supervise your health care for a number of years, there is much the doctor needs to know about you.

A typical history begins with a simple discussion of what may be troubling you at the moment. If you do have a complaint, the doctor will want you to describe your symptoms, how long you have had them, and how you noticed them developing. Then there is a probing of your past history, often a chronology from childhood until now. You will be asked about any chronic illnesses you may have, treatments you receive regularly, medicines you take, corrective devices you use.

Because some diseases are hereditary, the doctor will want to know about the health of your parents and grandparents, sisters and brothers. Then there is a long litany of questions that probes for information about allergies, diseases you have had, immunizations, operations, accidents, and injuries. There are personal questions:

What do you do for a living and what do you do in your leisure time? Do you smoke, drink, diet? Are you satisfied with your life? With your sex life? Are you worried, unhappy, or depressed?

You will be questioned about the functioning of all your body parts and systems, and you will be asked if you have noticed anything that seems unusual or has caused you concern. The more detailed and precise you can be about all this, the more the doctor has to work with when it comes to analyzing the state of your health.

What Makes You Qualified to Write a Medical History?

If you have ever filled out a medical questionnaire for an insurance company or on a first visit to a new doctor, you probably recall that you supplied most of the information yourself while your doctor had only a few questions to answer based on a brief medical examination. Despite the brief participation of a doctor, however, these questionnaires are quite reliable for health-screening purposes, and the reason they are reliable is that you are the world's leading expert on your own medical history. You are, in fact, the *only* person with a detailed knowledge of what has been happening to your body over the years; you know most about the family you were born into and you know most about the environment and social atmosphere in which your body must function.

Good doctors are expert at taking medical histories, but this simply means they have highly developed interviewing skills in the medical field rather than detailed knowledge of any one individual. Probing for special information in specific situations, organizing and analyzing information, and drawing medical conclusions—all of which require a physician's training and experience—come *after* you have supplied the bulk of the necessary medical history.

Why You Should Keep a Medical History and Personal Health Record

There are several major weaknesses in medical histories taken in the doctor's office. First, considering the level of pressure in many busy medical offices, there isn't always time to search your memory for things that happened years ago. And memories are fallible; it just isn't possible to remember all your past illnesses, treatments, and inoculations.

Many doctor-kept histories are taken when you are ill, because most people see a doctor only in times of sickness and distress. Histories taken at such times are full of bias and inaccuracies. Often, changes in your body and its functioning are more significant than signs, symptoms, and even test results at any one time on any one visit to a doctor's office. Increases in blood pressure, weight gain or loss, changing vision, changes in the texture of the breasts, changes in your skin, and changes in the operation of your digestive system are all of the utmost medical importance, and they are all more apparent to you, if you have been tracking your health, than they are at any one time to an examining physician.

Our new consciousness of occupational dangers and environmental pollution has made many people wish they had begun keeping health records many years ago. Chemicals, industrial dirt and dust, radiation, and drugs taken during pregnancy can all prove dangerous years after exposure to them. Without records, people often forget they have been exposed to these dangers or they are totally unaware that they have been exposed to a dangerous combination of elements. And without records to provide a clue, diagnosis of resulting ailments is often difficult and sometimes impossible.

Finally, we are a highly mobile society. Most people can recall treatment by a dozen or more doctors, often in medical facilities scattered across the country; and while medical records can be transferred from one doctor to another, few of us ever bother to have it done. It is a slow, tedious process, and if a medical emergency arises, there is certainly no time to write or call around to gather essential facts.

Thousands of times every day, throughout the country, patients turn up at the emergency receiving room of a hospital where the first person they meet is a doctor who is an absolute stranger. This physician knows nothing about them, their medical difficulties, the state of their body systems, their allergies, or their blood chemistry. Yet he or she must take immediate action. Under such circumstances diagnoses can be made more quickly and proper treatment prescribed more accurately when a medical history is available. Even in nonemergency medical situations, both time and money can be saved and medical treatment can be more satisfactory when the attending physician has a medical history and health record to work from.

How to Get Started

Just the thought of assembling all the data that goes into a medical history may seem overwhelming at first, but it's not that difficult to do. You can set down most of the basic facts in an hour or so and then gather other information as it is convenient. It could be the most important bit of work you've ever done for yourself and your family. All the questions you need to answer for a complete medical history and health record can be found in the following pages. To get started, do the easiest things first: name, birth date, place of birth, address, and telephone number. Once begun, the information will seem to pour forth, begging to be recorded.

Writing a medical history and personal health record makes a fascinating and educational family project when parents and children work together. In addition to creating valuable health documents that will serve each family member for a lifetime, you will have an opportunity to teach children about their bodies, discuss health problems and sex and sexuality, and expose hidden fears that may not come to light otherwise.

When compiling medical histories as a family project, each family member should have his or her own record. If you are computer-oriented, you can set up a computer file for each member of the family. A loose-leaf binder is even handier. Use the kind that has pocket pages you can use to keep copies of prescriptions, bills, and printed treatment instructions.

There is no special way to proceed as long as you do a thorough job and furnish all the information you can. Here are some tips that will help:

1. Do what is easiest for you first, then go back and fill in information that may require a little digging in your memory or inquiries among other members of the family.

2. Some information may have to be obtained from a doctor: total cholesterol and cholesterol ratios, blood type, blood pressure if you don't take it yourself, and so on. If you have had a recent physical examination, call the doctor's office and ask for the information you need. The office assistant can give it to you. If you haven't had a recent examination, this will give you a good excuse to do it now, and be sure to get all the information you need for your record from the doctor or the doctor's assistant at the time of your examination.

3. If you have moved or changed doctors and valuable records are scattered about the country, write for them. Some hospitals and doctors may not want to send information directly to you, so arrange to have it sent to your local doctor. If you have lost the address of a doctor or other health facility, local libraries have telephone books from all over the country that you can use to find it. Libraries also have national directories of doctors and hospitals you can use. Ask the reference

librarian in any medium-sized library. Most hospitals have libraries with national directories and most of them will help you find the information you need.

4. You can get much of the information called for from self-testing.

5. Some information has to be updated regularly. Be sure to do this as often as indicated.

The Contents of Your Medical History and Health Record

Who You Are

Begin your record as you would any other with your name, the date, and your occupation. Tell anything about yourself that explains who you are: married, single, children, your interests in life, and so on. Then list the following: date of birth, birthplace, race, body temperature, blood type, and Rh factor.

Your date of birth is important because your body is different at different times of your life and your health hazards are different. Birthplace and race are important because people of different races and from different countries are often genetically and culturally different in ways that can affect health.

Take your temperature several different times when you are well to record what is a normal body temperature for you. The well-known 98.6°F is not normal for everyone. Blood type and Rh factor are characteristics that are important to know for many medical procedures and during pregnancy.

Family History

On your family history page, tell what you can about serious chronic illnesses and ages and causes of death among your closest blood relatives. The only nonblood relative you should include is your spouse; chronic illness in a husband or wife may provide important information that is relevant for the rest of the family.

Begin with your father, mother, sisters and brothers, children, and spouse. Include blood-related aunts and uncles but omit cousins. Tell whether each is still alive, the age at death, and the cause of death if you know it. Inquire among family members to get information you don't know yourself. If any of your relatives have or have had chronic ailments such as asthma, migraine headaches, diabetes, allergies, and so on, list this information.

Immunization Records

Immunization records are often required for school, for certain jobs, and for foreign travel. If you are injured, the doctor will want to know when you had your last tetanus shot. Most people can't remember. Keep this record up-to-date and file any certificates in a place where they can be found easily when needed. The pocket pages of a loose-leaf binder are ideal for this, or keep a special file folder if you have a reliable filing system in your home. You will probably have to ask your doctor for some of this information when you start your health history because inoculations seem to be the easiest thing to forget.

Weight Tracking

It is no accident that the first dreaded procedure you must undergo whenever you visit a doctor is the weigh-in. Excess weight is so often a factor in heart and artery disease, stroke, diabetes, gallbladder problems, and other chronic diseases that the doctor has to know where you stand in this regard. Weight gain or weight loss over a period of time also provides significant information.

1. Head the page with what your weight was at age twenty as a basis for compar-

ison. Children usually gain height and weight along rather definite growth curves. This information can be provided by your doctor. If a child falls off his or her growth curve by any appreciable amount, this is important information to tell your doctor.

2. Weigh yourself once a month (or once a week if you are trying to gain or lose weight) and record the date and weight in your health record. Significant weight changes should be discussed with your doctor.

3. Record what you consider an ideal weight for you. Check with your doctor if you're

Maximum Recommended Weights

(Height without shoes, weight without clothing)

Men		Women	
5′ 1″	138	4′ 8″	110
5′ 2″	141	4′ 9″	113
5′ 3″	145	4′ 10″	116
5′ 4″	149	4′ 11″	120
5′ 5″	153	5′ 0″	123
5′ 6″	158	5′ 1″	126
5′ 7″	163	5′ 2″	129
5′ 8″	168	5′ 3″	132
5′ 9″	172	5′ 4″	136
5′ 10″	176	5′ 5″	139
5′ 11″	181	5′ 6″	143
6′ 0″	186	5′ 7″	147
6′ 1″	191	5′ 8″	151
6′ 2″	196	5′ 9″	155
6′ 3″	201	5′ 10″	160
6′ 4″	206	5′ 11″	165
6′ 5″	212	6′ 0″	170

not sure. Also record the percent you are under or over the maximum. People with a naturally slender build will be perfectly fine weighing less than is shown on the chart. You should not weigh much more, however, even if you have a husky build.

$$\frac{pounds\ over\ or\ under}{recommended\ maximum} = \begin{array}{l} percent\ over \\ or\ under \end{array}$$

Blood Pressure and Cholesterol Levels

These are two pieces of information that change even more than your weight, and if they change significantly you should find out why and what you can do about it.

Take your blood pressure once a month and record the results with the date. If there is a change from what you consider your normal blood pressure, take it at different times during the day: when you are rested and not stressed, after doing some average chore, and again after moderate exercise.

If your cholesterol levels are under control, your doctor will probably not want to check it more than every couple of years. If you have a problem, it should be checked more often. As you get the results of your cholesterol test, record it in your health record with the date. Record the HDL ratio as well as total cholesterol. The HDL ratio is

$$\frac{Total\ cholesterol}{HDL\ cholesterol}$$

Drugs and Alcohol Use

Keep track of the following information. If your habits change, record the change and the date.

1. Daily caffeine consumption in number of six-ounce servings, including coffee, tea, and cola drinks.

2. Daily alcohol consumption in one-ounce servings of eighty-proof spirits and six-ounce glasses of wine or beer. (A bottle or mug of beer is twelve ounces.)

3. Describe your smoking habits or other use of tobacco. If you have quit, say when.

4. List any illegal drugs you use. Describe the quantity and frequency of use.

5. List over-the-counter drugs you use regularly. Include antacids, headache or pain pills, sleeping aids, diet pills, laxatives, etc. List the frequency of use and the quantities you use.

6. List vitamins and supplements you use: quantities, dose size, and frequency.

Prescription Drugs

Make a record of drugs your doctor has prescribed. List the date, name of the drug, the potency, how often and for how long you took the drug, and in what quantity. Note why you took the drug and what the results of taking it were. You will also list prescribed drugs and how they worked for you in another section where you track ailments you have been treated for. But it is a good idea to keep a separate list where the doctor can see at a glance all the drugs you have taken and how they have affected you.

Special Diets

Describe any special diet you have been on whether prescribed by a doctor, on your own initiative, or as part of a commercial weight-control program. Tell how long and how carefully you followed the diet and what the results were.

Allergies

Make a list of substances you are allergic to and how they affect you. Include foods, drugs, cosmetics, animals, household substances, insect bites, etc. Describe any desensitizing treatments you have had and how well they worked. Record events of serious allergic reactions with their dates and treatment.

Occupational Health Hazards

List any possible health hazards you may be exposed to in your present job and any you may have been exposed to in the past. Include anything you may be suspicious of even if you have been assured that there is or was no danger. In addition to obvious physical hazards such as dangerous machinery, heights, weights, etc., possible occupational hazards include the following: all forms of radiation, odors, dusts of all kinds, unusual postures, chemicals, loud noises, repetitive motions, and stress and anxiety.

Emotional Health

Take a good inward look at yourself and answer the following questions. Review your answers from time to time to see if they have changed. Your emotional health is important information your doctor should know about, because stress levels can affect how your body functions and reacts to many ailments.

1. Explain what you think of your life in general: satisfactory, boring, too stressful, unhappy, etc. You might want to write a short paragraph to explain your feelings.

2. Everyone worries. What do you worry about most? Money, job, children, sex, relationships?

3. Do you cry easily, feel inferior or worthless, feel anxious or upset frequently, feel depressed, feel afraid for no reason?

4. Have you considered or attempted suicide?

5. Do you have difficulty sleeping? If yes, explain your sleep habits and patterns: when you go to bed, whether you take naps, whether you use tranquilizers or sleeping pills, how and where you sleep, whether you regularly eat or exercise before bedtime, whether you take caffeine pills or other stimulants during the day.

6. Are you argumentative, belligerent, impatient? Do you feel you are often picked on unfairly? Are you frequently "antsy" and constantly want to be doing something other than what you are doing?

Exercise Record

Keep separate pages or a separate computer file to record what you do for exercise.

1. Record the things you do *regularly* for exercise.

2. Record your resting pulse rate and your pulse after you have exercised vigorously. Describe the exercise and the length of time you did it before taking your pulse.

3. Record any adverse reactions to exercise.

4. If you are in a regular exercise program, record the progress you are making: distances walked or jogged, laps swum, aerobic workouts, and so on.

5. Comment on any improvements you notice in your health and well-being: weight loss, slower pulse, more endurance, better mental attitude, etc.

Record of Physical Examinations, Illnesses, and Treatments

Your doctor keeps extensive records and comments in your file describing the findings of each physical examination, diagnoses of illnesses, prescribed medicines and treatments, operations, test results, and so on. But it is just here that the doctor's records fall short and where you should fill in the gaps.

Your primary-care physician will have a record of what he or she has seen you for and what he or she has prescribed; if you have seen a specialist, there will be a file there, but the information may not get back to your primary-care doctor. If you have been in the hospital, those records will be separate from all the others.

You should keep a running record, as they happen, of every visit to the doctor, every illness treated, drugs prescribed, x-rays, tests, operations, and all the results of these visits and treatments. What is most important, and what your doctor won't have in his or her file, is how you responded to treatment, how you recovered from an operation, and whether you think the treatment helped you or not.

Keep visits to the doctor and a record of illnesses in the form of a running history or diary. Keep separate pages or files for chronic illnesses or major operations. For example, if you have diabetes or asthma, you should track your progress separately. If you have major surgery, you should keep a separate file that documents what went on and how the course of your recovery went. You should also have a place for questions you want to ask your doctor about your condition on your next follow-up visit.

Tracking Vision

The relevant records you want to keep about your vision are these: your visual acuity (how well you see at a distance and close up); your prescription if you use eyeglasses or contact lenses; and complaints you have about your ability to see and what has been done to correct the problems.

Visual Acuity. Distance vision is measured with the well-known fraction 20/something. The 20 is twenty feet, the accepted standard of "normal" vision for seeing the little letters on the eye chart. If the other side of the slanted line says 30, this means that a person with normal vision can see at thirty feet what you see at twenty. The figure 20/200 means the normal sighted person can see the big letter at the top of the chart from two hundred feet, but you have to read it from twenty feet, so your vision is quite limited compared with most people. Most authorities will let you drive an automobile without eyeglasses if your visual acuity is 20/30 or even 20/40, but you will probably feel more comfortable being corrected to 20/20.

Start a page in your health record that tracks your visual acuity. Record the date of each test with an eye chart and what the results were. Record the results both with and without your glasses if you wear them. Any change for the worse is significant and should be called to the attention of an eye doctor, especially if you are visiting a new doctor who doesn't have your previous records.

At about age forty, you will begin to notice that you have to hold small type farther and farther from your eyes to read it. Keep track of your near point as described in Chapter 4 on vision, and when it gets so far away that it's a nuisance, you will probably want to have reading glasses prescribed or added to your distance prescription as bifocal lenses.

Your Prescription. The prescription for eyeglasses or contact lenses an eye doctor gives you will look something like this:

	Spherical	Cylindrical	Axis
O.D.	−3.00	+1.50	180
O.S.	−2.50	+1.25	180
ADD	O.D. _____	O.S._____	

O.D. stands for *oculus dexter*, your right eye. O.S. stands for *oculus sinister*, your left eye. The only possible excuse for not saying right and left is that if you happen to run into a technician who can't read the words right and left, he or she should be able to recognize the abbreviations for the Latin words. It's the same reason that doctors use the Latin abbreviations *t.i.d.* for three times a day and *p.r.n.* for as needed. It adds a little cachet to things medical if you have difficulty understanding them.

The numbers indicate the power of the lenses in diopters that you require. A minus sign indicates a correction for nearsightedness. A plus sign indicates a correction for farsightedness. If there is a second set of numbers and an axis indicated, it means you have astigmatism; that is, your eyes focus differently in different planes of vision and the lenses will be ground to compensate for this.

The reason for keeping track of your prescriptions is to notice if there is any significant change—much larger numbers, for example—and you will want to ask why the change has occurred.

Problems and Treatments. Any difficulty you experience with seeing or any problems discovered by your doctor and the treatment you received should be recorded with the date and the results of the treatment.

Your Dental Record

One of the many things you surely won't remember about your health care is what the dentist did on your last visit. If you have changed dentists a number of times, as most people do, you will have no idea what has happened in the past, and dentists often want to know this information. (He or she will usually ask while there is a dental mirror and probe in your mouth.)

Keep a separate page or file to record your visits to the dentist. Explain briefly what was done and to which teeth. Date each entry. Refer to the chart of the teeth in Chapter 5 about the ears, nose, mouth, and throat and identify the teeth by number. If you ask, your dentist can give you a sheet from a pad that he or she keeps that shows all the teeth and how to record what work was done that day.

A Systems Review

A systems review is a battery of questions designed to uncover problems you may have with one or more of your body systems. A thorough annual physical examination should include a systems review, and in other times it did, before doctors fell under the time constraints of managed-care practices. If your doctor doesn't do a systems review, you should do it yourself about once a year and report any questionable findings.

Instructions: An answer of "yes" to any question hints at trouble and a doctor should be consulted. If you answer "yes" to a question, answer the follow-up questions to be able to describe the trouble more precisely to your doctor. Also refer to the chapter in this book that applies. Add your own comments whenever you feel they are necessary or helpful.

When you answer "no" to a question, move immediately to the next numbered question without bothering to answer the follow-up questions.

The Nervous System

1. Have you been having headaches recently?
   ❏ Yes   ❏ No

   Where are they located?
   ❏ Right side   ❏ Left side
   ❏ Front   ❏ Back
   ❏ All over

   Which of these describe your headache?
   ❏ Throbbing pain
   ❏ Constant pain
   ❏ Tight band
   ❏ Sudden, transient pain

   Other _____

   _____

   Do any of the following occur just before or with your headache?
   ❏ Blurred or swirly vision
   ❏ Other eye trouble
   ❏ Nausea or vomiting
   ❏ Stomach pain

2. Have you been having dizzy spells recently?
   ❏ Yes   ❏ No

   Do any of the following apply to your dizzy spells?
   ❏ They occur before meals.
   ❏ I bite my tongue.
   ❏ Eating something sweet helps.
   ❏ I shake all over.

Describe anything else that happens.

_____

_____

_____

_____

3. Have you fainted or had a convulsion
   in the past year or so?
   ❏ Yes   ❏ No
   ❏ I fainted.
   ❏ I fainted and had a convulsion.
   ❏ I had a convulsion.

   Describe what happened._____

   _____

   _____

   _____

   _____

4. Have you noticed a paralysis or
   weakness in any part of your body
   during the past year or so?
   ❏ Yes   ❏ No

   It was in my _____
   and I still have it.

   It was in my _____
   and it went away.

       ❏ It started suddenly.
       ❏ It came on gradually.

5. Have you had any numbness or
   tingling in your arms or legs lately?
   ❏ Yes   ❏ No

   Describe the feeling. _____

   _____

   _____

   _____

   _____

   Is there any special time when the feel-

   ing occurs? _____

   _____

   _____

   _____

6. Have you had any problems in the
   areas listed below?
   ❏ Yes   ❏ No
   ❏ Speech difficulty
   ❏ Trembling hands
   ❏ Trouble with fine movements,
      such as handwriting or buttoning
      clothes
   ❏ Memory loss

7. Have you been knocked unconscious
   in the past year?
   ❏ Yes   ❏ No
   ❏ I was really out cold.
   ❏ I was really just down
      and dizzy.

How did it happen? _____

_____

Skin

8. Do you have any problems with your skin, hair, or scalp? Read the following list before you decide.
   - ❏ Yes   ❏ No
   - ❏ Unusually dry, itchy skin
   - ❏ Pimples or boils
   - ❏ Rashes or hives
   - ❏ Eczema
   - ❏ Unusual reaction to sun
   - ❏ A nonhealing sore*
   - ❏ A changing mole*
   - ❏ Athlete's foot or other fungal infection

_____
Do not put off showing these to a physician.

Eyes

9. Do you have any trouble with your eyes or your ability to see clearly that is not corrected by wearing glasses? Read the following list before you decide.
   - ❏ Yes   ❏ No
   - ❏ Poor or dim vision not corrected by glasses
   - ❏ Narrow field of vision (like looking through a tunnel)
   - ❏ Double vision
   - ❏ Red or watery eyes
   - ❏ Burning or itching
   - ❏ Bulging or pop eyes
   - ❏ Whites of eyes quite yellow
   - ❏ Eye pain
   - ❏ Light flashes

   - ❏ Large drifting objects
   - ❏ Unusual sensitivity to light

10. Do you sometimes see spots before your eyes?
    - ❏ Yes   ❏ No
    - ❏ I see spots when I bend down.
    - ❏ I see spots when I stand up suddenly.
    - ❏ I see spots when I have a headache.
    - ❏ I see spots at other times. Explain.

    _____

    _____

Ears, Nose, Mouth, Throat, and Neck

11. Have you recently had any of the ear problems listed below?
    - ❏ Yes   ❏ No
    - ❏ Running or infected ears
    - ❏ Itchy ears
    - ❏ Difficulty hearing
    - ❏ Earaches
    - ❏ Buzzing or ringing noises

12. Have you recently had any of the nose problems listed below?
    - ❏ Yes   ❏ No
    - ❏ Frequent nosebleeds
    - ❏ Frequent runny nose or colds
    - ❏ Change in sense of smell
    - ❏ Sores in the nose
    - ❏ Frequent sneezing
    - ❏ Deformed nose
    - ❏ Sinus trouble
    - ❏ It has become red and veiny.

13. Have you had trouble with your mouth lately?
    ❏ Yes   ❏ No
    ❏ Toothaches or sensitivity
    ❏ Frequently have sores
    ❏ Bleeding gums
    ❏ Frequent trouble with
      my tongue. It doesn't
      feel right.

14. Has your voice become hoarse? Changed tone?
    ❏ Yes   ❏ No
    ❏ Hoarseness comes and goes.
    ❏ I always seem to be hoarse.

    Describe any changes in your voice.

    _____

    _____

15. Do you have any swollen glands or other lumps in your neck?
    ❏ Yes   ❏ No

    If yes, describe what you have. _____

    _____

    _____

16. Have you been having trouble with your throat or tonsils?
    ❏ Yes   ❏ No
    ❏ Throat dryness
    ❏ Difficulty swallowing
    ❏ Frequent sore throat
    ❏ Tonsillitis

Describe any other problems. _____

_____

_____

_____

17. Have you been coughing a lot?
    ❏ Yes   ❏ No

    The cough is
    ❏ worse in the morning
    ❏ worse afternoons and evenings
    ❏ about the same all day and night

    What do you cough up?
    ❏ Nothing
    ❏ Yellow-white material
    ❏ Green material
    ❏ Red or black material
    ❏ Frothy material

18. Have you coughed up blood in the past year?
    ❏ Yes   ❏ No

    If yes, when? _____

    _____

    _____

19. Have you had difficulty breathing recently?
    ❏ Yes   ❏ No
    ❏ Shortness of breath
    ❏ Wheezing sounds
    ❏ Hard to breathe

Describe any other difficulties. _____

_____

_____

When does the difficulty occur?
- ❏ When climbing stairs
- ❏ When exercising
- ❏ All the time
- ❏ If seasonally, when? _____

_____

Tell of any other times not mentioned.

_____

_____

20. Do you sometimes wake up at night because you are short of breath or you have difficulty breathing?
- ❏ Yes   ❏ No

How many pillows do you use when

you sleep? _____

21. Do you often wake up at night and find yourself soaked in sweat?
- ❏ Yes   ❏ No

If yes, how often does this happen?

_____

_____

Chest Pain

22. Have you been having pains in your chest lately?
- ❏ Yes   ❏ No
- ❏ I seem to have hurt my chest or my shoulder.
- ❏ It just started and I don't know why.

What is the pain like?
- ❏ Sharp
- ❏ Dull
- ❏ Squeezing

Where is the pain?
- ❏ It seems to be inside.
- ❏ It seems to be outside around the ribs.

How bad is the pain?
- ❏ Not too bad
- ❏ Moderate
- ❏ Very bad

Where is the pain located, exactly?
- ❏ On the right
- ❏ On the left
- ❏ In the middle
- ❏ In the back or shoulders
- ❏ All over

When you feel the pain, how long does it last?
- ❏ A few seconds
- ❏ A few minutes
- ❏ Hours
- ❏ Several days
- ❏ I have it most of the time.

When does the pain occur?
- ❏ Generally at night or in bed
- ❏ Generally during the day
- ❏ Mostly when I exercise
- ❏ When I'm resting
- ❏ No special time

When you have chest pain, do you also have one or more of the following?
- ❏ Pain in the left arm
- ❏ Pain in the jaw or neck
- ❏ Pain in the shoulder

Do any of these make your chest pain better?
- ❏ Exercise
- ❏ Medicine
- ❏ Eating
- ❏ Rest

If medicine makes it better, what kind?

_____

_____

Do any of these make your chest pain worse?
- ❏ Exercise
- ❏ Food
- ❏ Rest
- ❏ Coffee

If something else, describe it. _____

_____

_____

When you have chest pain, do you have any of these other things?
- ❏ Sweating
- ❏ Weakness
- ❏ Feeling of nausea
- ❏ I feel my heart beating.

23. Does your heart sometimes seem to beat in an unusual way?
- ❏ Yes   ❏ No
- ❏ It beats irregularly, skips a beat.
- ❏ It beats very slowly.
- ❏ It beats very rapidly.

How often does this happen? _____

_____

_____

Digestion

24. Do you have any of the following problems with your digestion?
- ❏ Yes   ❏ No
- ❏ Fatty or fried foods disagree with me.
- ❏ I frequently have indigestion.
- ❏ My digestion is just plain bad.

What foods seem to disagree with you?

_____

_____

_____

25. Has your abdomen or belly gotten abnormally swollen or enlarged?
    ❑ Yes   ❑ No

    If yes, how do you know? _____

    _____

    _____

If you can locate it precisely, describe

where it is._____

_____

_____

26. Do you have abdominal (belly) pain, distress, or discomfort?
    ❑ Yes   ❑ No
    ❑ Pain
    ❑ Distress
    ❑ Heartburn
    ❑ Burning under the breastbone
    ❑ Something else? _____

    When does this discomfort occur?
    ❑ Before meals
    ❑ After meals
    ❑ At night
    ❑ During the day

    If some other times, when?_____

    _____

    _____

    Where would you say the pain or discomfort is located?
    ❑ Mostly on the left side
    ❑ Mostly on the right side
    ❑ Mostly in the middle
    ❑ It's all over.
    ❑ It spreads to my back.

Do you take something for your problem?
    ❑ Yes   ❑ No

If yes, what? (Antacid, laxative, food or

drink, something else) _____

_____

_____

27. Have you been vomiting frequently during the past year?
    ❑ Yes   ❑ No

If yes, what does the material that comes up look like?
    ❑ Like pieces of food just eaten
    ❑ Like coffee grounds
    ❑ Like something else (describe it)

_____

_____

_____

_____

28. Do you have any of the following problems?
    - ❏ Yes   ❏ No
    - ❏ Frequent belching
    - ❏ Frequent hiccups
    - ❏ Food sticks on the way down

29. During the past year, did the whites of your eyes turn yellow? Did your skin ever turn yellow? Were you told you have jaundice?
    - ❏ Yes   ❏ No
    - ❏ Whites of eyes were yellow.
    - ❏ Skin was yellow.
    - ❏ Skin and eyes were yellow.
    - ❏ I had jaundice.

30. Have you had trouble with bowel movements recently?
    - ❏ Yes   ❏ No
    - ❏ Diarrhea frequently
    - ❏ Frequently constipated
    - ❏ Pain with bowel movements
    - ❏ Unable to hold bowel movements long enough to get to a toilet
    - ❏ I take a laxative frequently.

31. Have your stools been an unusual color or odor during the past year?
    - ❏ Yes   ❏ No
    - ❏ Black or tarlike
    - ❏ Red or blood-smeared
    - ❏ Unusually foul-smelling
    - ❏ Very light, almost white

32. Have you had any bleeding from your rectum?
    - ❏ Yes   ❏ No

33. Do you think you have hemorrhoids (piles)?
    - ❏ Yes   ❏ No

    If yes, what makes you think so? ____

    _____

    _____

Urination

34. Do you have any of the following problems with urination?
    - ❏ Yes   ❏ No
    - ❏ Can't always hold urine
    - ❏ Dribbling
    - ❏ Bed-wetting
    - ❏ Difficulty starting flow
    - ❏ Sometimes pass urine when I cough or sneeze
    - ❏ Pain or burning with urination

35. Do you get up at night to urinate?
    - ❏ Yes   ❏ No

    If yes, how often each night? _____

    _____

36. Have you passed red or bloody urine during the past year?
    - ❏ Yes   ❏ No

37. Have you noticed any change in the force of the stream of urine during the past year?
    - ❏ Yes   ❏ No

38. Have you ever been told (or found by self-testing) that you have sugar or other substances in your urine?

    ❏ Yes   ❏ No

    If yes, what substances have been

    found? _____

    _____

    _____

39. Do you seem always thirsty and take large quantities of fluid to relieve your thirst?

    ❏ Yes   ❏ No

The Male Reproductive System

40. Have you had any difficulties with erections recently?

    ❏ Yes   ❏ No
    ❏ It is difficult to have an erection at all.
    ❏ Erections are often painful.

41. Have you had a sore on your genitals?

    ❏ Yes   ❏ No

42. Have you noticed any change in your testicles?

    ❏ Yes   ❏ No
    ❏ They seem to be getting smaller.
    ❏ They seem to be getting larger.
    ❏ I think a lump is developing in there.
    ❏ They have become tender.

43. Do you think you are sterile (unable to father children), or do you have reason to be certain of it?

    ❏ Yes   ❏ No
    ❏ I've had a sterilization operation.
    ❏ I have tried but have been unable to have children.

    If a physician has told you so, explain

    why. _____

    _____

44. Do you have reason to suspect you should be examined or tested for venereal disease?

    ❏ Yes   ❏ No

    If yes, explain why you think so. ____

    _____

    _____

    _____

45. Do you think you may have prostate trouble?

    ❏ Yes   ❏ No

    If yes, what makes you think so? ____

    _____

    _____

    _____

46. Have you developed a hernia
    (rupture) in the past year?
    ❑ Yes   ❑ No

    If yes, what makes you think so? ____

    _____

    _____

    _____

47. Have you had any swollen glands or
    other lumps in your groin?
    ❑ Yes   ❑ No

The Female Reproductive System

48. Have you had a miscarriage or
    spontaneous abortion or an elective
    abortion?
    ❑ Yes   ❑ No
    ❑ Miscarriage or spontaneous
       abortion
    ❑ Elective abortion
    ❑ Attended by a physician
    ❑ Not attended by a physician

49. Have your periods changed during the
    past year?
    ❑ Yes   ❑ No
    ❑ They've become lighter.
    ❑ They've become heavier.
    ❑ They are longer.
    ❑ They are shorter.
    ❑ They are irregular.
    ❑ They always were irregular but
       now more than usual.
    ❑ Pain with periods

❑ Bleeding between periods
❑ Other change (explain)

_____

_____

_____

50. Are you generally nervous or tense
    before your periods start?
    ❑ Yes   ❑ No

51. Do you use any kind of birth control?
    ❑ Yes   ❑ No

    What kind of birth control do you use?

    _____

    Do you have any problems related to

    your mode of birth control? _____

    _____

    _____

52. Have you had any unusual vaginal
    discharge during the past year?
    ❑ Yes   ❑ No

    If yes, describe it and how long it

    lasted._____

    _____

    _____

53. Have you been having pain during sexual intercourse?

    ❑ Yes   ❑ No

54. Do you have reason to suspect you should be examined or tested for venereal disease?

    ❑ Yes   ❑ No

    If yes, explain why you think so. ____

    _____

    _____

55. Do you have any pain in your breasts?

    ❑ Yes   ❑ No

56. Do you have a discharge or bleeding from the nipples?

    ❑ Yes   ❑ No

57. Have you noticed a lump in either breast?

    ❑ Yes   ❑ No

    If yes, describe the exact location and what you feel. (See Chapter 10, "Tests and Observations of the Reproductive Organs," for a description of breast self-examination.)

    _____

    _____

    _____

    _____

58. Have you noticed that one or both of your nipples seem to be retracting into the breast?

    ❑ Yes   ❑ No

59. Does the skin of either breast seem to be puckering or dimpling?

    ❑ Yes   ❑ No

General Questions

60. Do you have any problems or complaints with your sex life?

    ❑ Yes   ❑ No

    If yes, explain. _____

    _____

    _____

61. Have you become unusually pale recently, or do you have some reason to believe you are anemic?

    ❑ Yes   ❑ No

    If yes, tell about it. _____

    _____

    _____

62. Do you notice bruises about your body that appear without apparent reason?

    ❑ Yes   ❑ No

    Where do they occur?_____

    _____

Do they persist or quickly disappear?   When do they occur? _____

_____   _____

_____   _____

63. Are you generally uncomfortable at
    the same temperature as most other
    people seem comfortable?
    ❏ Yes   ❏ No
    ❏ I'm generally hotter.
    ❏ I'm generally colder.

64. Are you unusually tired or sluggish a
    good deal of the time?
    ❏ Yes   ❏ No

65. Do you notice any of the following
    occurring?
    ❏ Yes   ❏ No
    ❏ Eyes bulging or developing a
      wide-eyed, pop-eyed appearance
    ❏ A swelling in the neck
    ❏ Eating more than usual with no
      weight gain
    ❏ Jumpiness or unusual
      nervousness

66. Have you been having pains or
    cramps in your legs or feet?
    ❏ Yes   ❏ No

    Where do you have the pains? _____

    _____

    _____

67. Have you noticed that your ankles
    have been swelling?
    ❏ Yes   ❏ No
    ❏ Usually swollen in the evening
    ❏ They swell only after I stand a
      long time.
    ❏ They swell only in hot weather.
    ❏ Swollen nearly all the time
    ❏ Other times (when?) _____

68. Have you recently developed
    varicose veins?
    ❏ Yes   ❏ No

69. Do you have swollen glands or other
    lumps in your armpits?
    ❏ Yes   ❏ No

70. Have your fingers or toes been getting
    very white frequently and easily?
    ❏ Yes   ❏ No

71. Have you had pain, stiffness, or
    swelling in any of your joints?
    ❏ Yes   ❏ No
    ❏ On and off
    ❏ All the time

    Where? _____

    _____

    _____

72. Do you have any trouble with your
back or neck?
❏ Yes   ❏ No

If yes, describe it. _____

_____

_____

_____

73. Have any of the following things
happened to you recently?
❏ Yes   ❏ No
❏ Tenderness or swelling on
a bone
❏ Lump or swelling in a muscle
❏ Unusually stiff or sore muscles
❏ Muscle seems to be getting
smaller or weaker.

Explain what you have felt. _____

_____

_____

_____

Feelings and Emotions

74. Do you often feel afraid without
cause, panicky, or frightened?
❏ Yes   ❏ No

75. Read the following list of statements.
Do any of them apply to you?
❏ Yes   ❏ No

❏ My marriage is not very happy.
❏ My children bother me.
❏ There is more tension at home
than I can bear.
❏ I always worry about money.
❏ I often can't control my temper.
❏ Things never go right for me.
❏ I'm too shy with people.
❏ I'm just no good.

76. Are you often depressed? Do you
cry easily or feel like crying much
of the time?
❏ Yes   ❏ No

77. Have you thought seriously about
suicide in the past year?
❏ Yes   ❏ No

While there is illness enough in the world, for most of us, for the vast majority of the time, all of our body systems work together so well that we are barely aware of them, with the exception of occasional complaints that come and go. But it's only prudent to keep an eye on this marvelous machinery as you would on a dependable car you intend to keep in service for many years to come. Most of the time it purrs down the highway without your having to worry about the intricacies of the computer-controlled carburetor or how the automatic transmission works, but every once in a while you need to check fluid levels, tire-tread wear, and how the brake pads are faring, and from time to time you have to find out what a new, strange noise is all about.

It is, after all, your primary responsibility to take care of yourself and be aware of problems you need to bring to your doctor's attention, just as it is your primary responsibility to know when there is something wrong with your car that needs to be looked at by a mechanic. If you are conscientious about keeping track of your body systems, watching for changes from the relatively smooth functioning you are used to, you can catch problems before they become serious and you will be healthier and happier for it. We hope we have helped to show you how to do this.